RENAL AND UROLOGIC DISORDERS

HYPOSPADIAS

RISK FACTORS, EPIDEMIOLOGY AND SURGICAL OUTCOMES

RENAL AND UROLOGIC DISORDERS

Additional books in this series can be found on Nova's website under the Series tab.

Additional e-books in this series can be found on Nova's website under the e-book tab.

RENAL AND UROLOGIC DISORDERS

HYPOSPADIAS

RISK FACTORS, EPIDEMIOLOGY AND SURGICAL OUTCOMES

DANIEL H. PRESTON
EDITOR

NOVA BIOMEDICAL

New York

Library of Congress Cataloging-in-Publication Data

ISBN: 978-1-63482-023-3
Library of Congress Control Number: 2015930587

Published by Nova Science Publishers, Inc. † New York

Contents

Preface

Hypospadias is recognized as one the most common congenital malformations in male newborns, resulting in an abnormal opening of urethral meatus. It is regarded as a multifactorial disorder in which interactions between genetics, maternal and environmental factors lead to hypoplastic development of the ventral side of the penis, either dependently or in an interaction with other factors. This book discusses the risk factors of hypospadias. It also examines the epidemiology and surgical outcomes of hypospadias.

Chapter 1 – This chapter is a review of the published literature on the descriptive epidemiology of hypospadias. The authors will summarize associations between hypospadias and familial characteristics that have been included in published descriptive epidemiology studies, especially focusing on results from large population-based studies. These characteristics include geographical differences; infant, maternal, and paternal demographic and socioeconomic factors; and other variables available from vital records, such as parity, plurality, and race/ethnicity. Although the prevalence of hypospadias has been reported to be increasing in the 1970s and soon after, it seems to have stabilized in recent years, and the authors will also review reported trends in the prevalence of hypospadias over time. Similarities and differences between reported associations with each characteristic from descriptive epidemiology studies will be compared across studies. For example, over twenty studies have reported positive associations between multiple gestation pregnancies and hypospadias. Several characteristics have been associated with hypospadias in descriptive epidemiologic studies that may suggest endocrine-related pathways and mechanisms, such as parity, plurality, and body mass index, and the authors will review this evidence and discuss the implications of these findings (e.g., maternal characteristics that predict aberrant estrogen levels may be involved in hypospadias etiology). The authors will briefly compare associations that have been reported in descriptive epidemiologic studies of hypospadias to associations that have been reported in descriptive epidemiologic studies of other male genital defects. This chapter will also include a review of study design and methodological issues in these descriptive epidemiologic studies of hypospadias, including overall strengths and limitations, and there will be a discussion of future directions and conclusions.

Chapter 2 – Hypospadias is recognized as one the most common congenital malformations in male newborns, resulting in an abnormal opening of urethral meatus. It is regarded as a multifactorial disorder in which interactions between genetics, maternal and environmental factors lead to hypoplastic development of the ventral side of the penis, either dependently or in an interaction with other factors. Various studies have pointed to contributing factors and their association with development of hypospadias. In addition epidemiologic studies have described its epidemiologic patterns. In this chapter, the authors aim to summarize various epidemiological findings, mutations and the recognized genetic aspects of the malformation, as well as the known predisposing environmental factors. Some gene-gene and gene-environment interactions have been recognized which will be discussed. Finally, the tendency of each etiologic factor to result in different phenotypes will be described.

Chapter 3 – In the past several decades, numerous advances in the field of tissue engineering have been made towards the management of hypospadias and associated urethral defects. Reliable products for clinical use still remain elusive, however. Hypospadias affects approximately 0.3% of live births with current practice favoring early repair. With the advances in surgical approaches to hypospadias repair, such as the tubularized-incised plate, mid-shaft and distal variants rarely require supplemental tissue. In more proximal and perineal urethral defects, and especially in the case of the hypospadias cripple, however, patients may lack adequate, healthy local tissue for definitive repair. Ongoing research into the use of acellular matrix grafts and cell-seeded matrix grafts have produced promising results in animal models. Unfortunately, these grafts can be plagued by graft loss, graft contracture, stricture formation, and fistulization. Extensive additional research remains to evaluate the long-term biosafety and efficacy of these materials and to determine a reproducible and cost-effective means for their use in clinical practice.

Chapter 4 – Although fistula historically has been the most common complication in hypospadias surgery, with a frequency up to 11%, the incidence has decreased during the last 20 years to less than 5%. Rarely some small fistulas resolve spontaneously. Nonetheless, recurrence is still possible. Many solutions are available to decrease the incidence of fistula, such as use of better suture materials, microsurgical instruments, magnification, silicone catheters or stents, reliable postoperative dressing and vascularized island flaps to protect the neourethra the use of flaps to cover the neourethra has been shown to decrease the incidence. The authors report our experience to prevent and to repair urethrocutaneous fistula in hypospadias surgery.

Chapter 5 – *Introduction:* Elastosonography analyzes the variable elasticity of a tissue by recording the changes of RF pulses from a structure, before and after manual compression. The aim of this study is to apply the elastosonography on normal and hypospadic penis to verify the structural differences in tissues composition and stiffness. *Materials and Methods:* 60 subjects were enrolled, mean age 24 months: 38 patients on post-operative follow-up for distal hypospadia and 22 age-matched subjects as control group (11 patients waiting for surgery and 11 patients without hypospadias). Elastosonography recorded antero-posterior and transverse diameters of the cavernous corpora, urethral and corpus spongiosum diameters, elastographic index of elasticity of the corpus spongiosum. The latter was defined as soft, medium-hard or hard. The authors assigned the value 1 to soft tissue, 2 and 3 to medium-hard and hard respectively. All scan were performed at the base of the penis, as far as possible from the region involved in the surgical procedure. *Results:* Average antero-posterior and transverse diameters of the cavernous corpora were 4.2 mm (DS 0.83) and 6.5 mm (DS 1.12) for hypospadic group and 7.3 mm (DS 1.28) and 9.0 mm (DS 1.67) for control group. These data showed statistically significant difference between the two groups for both the diameters ($p<0.05$). Corpus spongiosum diameter was 1.9 (DS 0.33) for hypospadic group and 2.7 mm (DS 0.73) for control group ($p<0.05$). Less stiffness after surgery due to the chordee resection. Elastography showed a corpus spongiosum stiffness defined as medium-hard or hard in all cases of the pathologic group and soft in all the subjects of the control group ($p<0.05$). No significant difference was found for urethra diameter between the two groups. *Conclusions:* Elastosonography showed how the hypospadia anatomy is deeply altered, even in an anatomical area far from meatal abnormality: corpus spongiosum in hypospadic penis seems to be globally stiffer and less elastic. Moreover, cavernous corpora are less developed. These results could be used for pre-operative counseling. These preliminary results suggest the feasibility of the elastosonography for the evaluation of hypospadic penis. It could be useful during surgical plan to have a better definition of the calibers and quality of the tissues, especially in proximal hypospadia. The authors believe that this methodic could also be important during the early post-operative follow-up.

In: Hypospadias
Editor: Daniel H. Preston

ISBN: 978-1-63482-023-3

Chapter 1

Descriptive Epidemiology of Hypospadias

A. J. Agopian, PhD,[1*] S. Shahrukh Hashmi, MD PhD[2] and Anushuya Ramakrishnan[1]

[1]Division of Epidemiology, Human Genetics, and Environmental Sciences, University of Texas School of Public Health, Houston, TX, US
[2]Department of Pediatrics, University of Texas Medical School, Houston, TX, US

Abstract

This chapter is a review of the published literature on the descriptive epidemiology of hypospadias. We will summarize associations between hypospadias and familial characteristics that have been included in published descriptive epidemiology studies, especially focusing on results from large population-based studies. These characteristics include geographical differences; infant, maternal, and paternal demographic and socioeconomic factors; and other variables available from vital records, such as parity, plurality, and race/ethnicity. Although the prevalence of hypospadias has been reported to be increasing in the 1970s and soon after, it seems to have stabilized in recent years, and we will also review

[*] Address for correspondence: A.J. Agopian, Ph.D., University of Texas School of Public Health, 1200 Herman Pressler Dr., Houston, TX 77030, a.j.agopian@uth.tmc.edu

reported trends in the prevalence of hypospadias over time. Similarities and differences between reported associations with each characteristic from descriptive epidemiology studies will be compared across studies. For example, over twenty studies have reported positive associations between multiple gestation pregnancies and hypospadias. Several characteristics have been associated with hypospadias in descriptive epidemiologic studies that may suggest endocrine-related pathways and mechanisms, such as parity, plurality, and body mass index, and we will review this evidence and discuss the implications of these findings (e.g., maternal characteristics that predict aberrant estrogen levels may be involved in hypospadias etiology). We will briefly compare associations that have been reported in descriptive epidemiologic studies of hypospadias to associations that have been reported in descriptive epidemiologic studies of other male genital defects. This chapter will also include a review of study design and methodological issues in these descriptive epidemiologic studies of hypospadias, including overall strengths and limitations, and there will be a discussion of future directions and conclusions.

Introduction

Structural birth defects are a group of conditions that are common and costly, and these conditions have serious medical consequences. Approximately eight million infants are born with a major birth defect worldwide each year (~6% of infants) (Christianson et al., 2006). Of these, approximately three million die before age five, and another three million of the surviving infants experience life-long disabilities related to the birth defect (Christianson et al., 2006). Further, many affected individuals and/or their family members experience a profound psychosocial impact (Heller et al., 1985; Holmbeck and Devine, 2010). In the U.S., birth defects are the leading cause of childhood hospitalizations (Yoon et al., 1997) and the lifelong cost of birth defects for infants born in the U.S. each year is estimated to exceed six billion dollars (Centers for Disease Control and Prevention, 1995). Despite the substantial impact of birth defects at the individual-, family-, and society-levels, our understanding of the determinants of birth defects is limited. In the majority of affected individuals, the etiology is unknown.

Descriptive epidemiology focuses on describing the patterns of the distributions of health outcomes, typically with respect to factors related to personal, geographical, and temporal characteristics. When the etiology of a health outcome is not well-understood, descriptive epidemiology studies are often performed as a first step towards generating novel hypotheses about potential risk factors. Thus, descriptive epidemiology studies often precede analytic epidemiology studies, which typically evaluate specific risk factors more comprehensively than descriptive epidemiology studies (i.e., testing hypotheses about specific exposure-outcome relationships).

Further, in addition to evaluating trends that may provide insight into etiology, objectives of descriptive epidemiology also include identifying emerging health problems and providing data for efficient allocating of resources and health services.

Descriptive epidemiology has been a powerful tool for gaining insight into the etiology of birth defects. Descriptive characteristics that have been evaluated include characteristics of the infant/pregnancy (e.g., sex, plurality, birth year), mother/father (e.g., age, race/ethnicity, birthplace, education, parity), and family (e.g., family history of birth defects, residence location, income). Because birth defects as a group are heterogeneous with respect to etiology, individual types of birth defects (e.g., hypospadias) are often analyzed separately.

This chapter will discuss the descriptive epidemiology of one of the most common birth defects observed in males, hypospadias. Hypospadias is a defect in the penis, which involves the urethra opening on the underside of the penis instead of on the tip of the glans of the penis. This defect is often further classified based on the degree of severity (first-, second-, or third- degree), and there may be some etiologic heterogeneity across these subtypes.

In this chapter, we will summarize published research in this area; report on associations that have been identified by these studies; discuss the implications of these findings; and comment on study design, methodological issues, and future directions.

The scope of this review includes major maternal, infant, and familial characteristics that are frequently assessed in descriptive epidemiology studies, including pregnancy features, demographic and socio-economic factors, and common maternal conditions. It will not include a review of other factors such as medications, diet/behavioral factors, environmental/occupational exposures, genetic factors, or exposures/outcomes that occur after early pregnancy (e.g., gestational age or low birth weight at delivery).

Background on Epidemiologic Studies

One of the most important factors to consider when comparing results from the various epidemiologic reports on hypospadias is the methodologies of the studies that yielded the data. The different approaches adopted in these studies are often based on what may or may not be feasible for the researchers and, in turn, give rise to strengths and limitations that influence the reliability and validity of the dataset. Therefore, the strength of the evidence reported in the studies varies considerably based on differences in the study design, methodology, and analysis (Elwood, 2007; Jenicek, 2003). In the following sections, we will discuss such differences in descriptive studies of hypospadias.

Study Design

Many of the limitations observed in epidemiological studies of hypospadias are due to the relative rarity of the birth defect (<1% of males). Observational epidemiologic studies can be grouped into categories based on the temporal nature of the ascertained data.

Cohort studies (also called longitudinal or prospective studies) involve establishing a cohort of study subjects and following them prospectively over time until the outcome of interest occurs (Song and Chung, 2010). A major strength of a cohort study is the ability to definitively establish that the exposure of interest preceded the outcome. However, for rare outcomes, such as hypospadias, a considerably large cohort would have to be followed for a long period of time to provide a researcher with an adequate sample of individuals with hypospadias. Thus, prospective designs are not typically feasible for birth defects research. A special type of longitudinal study is the retrospective or historical cohort study. In these studies the investigator uses data sources that were collected at some point in the past and then "follows-up" on the cohort(s) via the records. Compared to other longitudinal studies, the fact that the data has already been collected is both a strength (prolonged recruitment and/or data collection period is not required) and a limitation (record source is required and only data that is already available can be used) in these historical cohorts. In retrospective case-control studies, individuals with and without the outcome of interest (cases and controls, respectively) are sampled and recruited, and past exposures for both groups are ascertained

(Song and Chung, 2010). Since the cases have already occurred, these studies are easier to administer in a relatively shorter amount of time to yield a sufficient sample size. A third group is cross-sectional studies wherein a snapshot of disease (and exposure if applicable) is taken at a fixed point in time. Most descriptive studies reporting on the prevalence of a disease or defect are cross-sectional in design. Although associations between "exposures" and an outcome can be reported in these studies, a causal relationship cannot be definitively established (Song and Chung, 2010).

There are other studies that employ designs that expand beyond classic epidemiologic study designs, such as some registry-based studies. For example, in many registry-based studies of hypospadias, data on cases were collected and prior exposure status was determined based on vital records or medical records rather than conducting interviews. These studies are retrospective in nature; however, the comparison group may be based on all live-births in the population, rather than control subjects. The majority of hypospadias studies have been case-control studies or registry-based studies that consider the entire population rather than a sample of controls.

Some studies have employed a "case-only" design, although this is not considered a "classic" epidemiologic study design. Under this approach, no unaffected subjects are considered; thus, there is no comparison group and it is therefore difficult to determine if any observed trends represent differences between affected subjects and the general population versus systematic error in the study. Results from such a study should generally be considered with skepticism.

Temporality of Exposure Assessment and Recall Bias

Retrospective studies and cross-sectional studies are, in some aspects, inferior to prospective studies by nature of the data collection process. In retrospective studies, since cases and controls are queried about exposures in the past, depending on the nature of the exposure and the time elapsed, there can be a differential degree of error in ascertainment of the exposure; this is known as recall bias. For example, the mother of a child with a birth defect may scrutinize her history of past exposures more than the mother of an unaffected child, and therefore may be more likely to correctly recall an exposure that occurred a year or longer in the past. Because of the long time period between early pregnancy (i.e., the relevant exposure period for hypospadias) and the time point at which hypospadias cases are ascertained by researchers (often months after delivery), recall bias is not a trivial concern. The level of recall bias is dependent on the variable being queried. For example, gender or ethnicity would not change over time and can be considered to present no issues of recall bias, regardless of when they are reported. Other factors, such as number of pregnancies, may also be in that same category since most women would be able to accurately report such factors. However, questions on diet or other environmental exposures may be harder to recall, especially if enough time has elapsed since the exposure. To gauge the quality of the publication, the reader must be cognizant of these biases and judge the validity and interpretation of the results in light of these limitations. Only a few longitudinal studies of hypospadias have been performed. To our knowledge, all of these have been a special subset of longitudinal studies known as the "retrospective cohort." In these studies, cases and controls are identified initially. The investigator then goes back to a time in the past, for example, 10 years prior to the birth of the child, and begins reviewing prospectively collected data that was ascertained over those 10 years. The feasibility of such study designs are dependent on the presence of data that was collected prospectively beginning from some point in the past. Therefore, it is not surprising that most of the retrospective cohort studies were performed in countries with socialized health care systems, where data from all encounters with the system are collected and stored in a central repository. Since the data is collected prospectively, albeit in the past, the issues of recall bias do not influence these studies.

Source of Study Subject Ascertainment: Population-based vs. Clinic-based Studies

The way in which hypospadias cases and unaffected subjects are selected is also an important consideration. The source of the study sample can influence who is included in the study and can potentially give rise to "selection bias." This bias occurs when a study participant is able to (consciously or not) select themselves into or out of a study in a non-random manner, and the potential for selection bias varies with the source of the data. A number of clinic-based studies on the epidemiology of hypospadias have been reported (Akin et al., 2011; Brouwers et al., 2010; Fredell et al., 2002; Ghirri et al., 2009; Giordano et al., 2010; Hussain et al., 2002; Mavrogenis et al., 2014; Morera et al., 2006; Nelson et al., 2005; Sun et al., 2009; van Rooij et al., 2013; Xu et al., 2014).

Table 1. Summary of key studies evaluating descriptive characteristics and hypospadias

Author (s)	Publication year	Study location	Cases (N)	Study Period	Population-based	Adjustment[A]	Non-syndromic[B]
Agopian et al.	2014	Texas	8,680	1999–2008	Yes	Yes	Yes
Aviles et al.	2014	Puerto Rico	279	2007-2010	Yes	Yes	No
Mavrogenis et al.	2014	Hungary	3,038	1980-1996	No	Yes	Yes
Nordenvall et al.	2014	Sweden	7,974	1973-2009	Yes	Yes	No
Winston et al.	2014	North Carolina	995	2003-2005	Yes	Yes	No
Woud et al.	2014	United States[C]	1,936	1997-2009	Yes	Yes	Yes
Xu et al.	2014	China	193	2003-2012	No	No	No
Marengo et al.	2013	Texas	4,546	2005-2008	Yes	Yes	No
van Rooij et al.	2013	Netherlands	405	1987-2006	No	Yes	Yes
Canon et al.	2012	Arkansas	1,455	1998-2007	Yes	Yes	No
Gill et al.	2012	United States[C]	1,466	1997-2007	Yes	Yes	No
Akin et al.	2011	Istanbul	34	2007-2008	No	No	No
Brouwers et al.	2010	Netherlands	305	1996-2004	No	Yes	No
Giordano et al.	2010	Italy	80	2005-2007	No	Yes	No
Jin et al.	2010	China	241	1993-2005	Yes	Yes	No
Nassar et al.	2010	Australia	1,202	1980-2000	Yes	Yes	No
Carlson et al.	2009	Nova Scotia	995	1980-2007	Yes	Yes	No
Fisch et al.	2009	New York	-[D]	1992-2005	Yes	No	No
Ghirri et al.	2009	Italy	234	2001-2004	No	Yes	No
Lund et al.	2009	Denmark	3,490	1977-2005	Yes	Yes	No
Sun et al.	2009	China	75	1998-2007	No	No	No
Akre et al.	2008	Denmark and Sweden	292	2000-2005	Yes	Yes	No
Correa et al.	2008	United States[C]	936	1997-2003	Yes	Yes	Yes
Brouwers et al.	2007	Netherlands	583	1987-1997	No	Yes	No
Carmichael et al.	2007	United States[C]	502	1997-2000	Yes	Yes	No
Meyer et al.	2006	Arkansas	354	1998-2002	Yes	Yes	No

Table 1. (Continued)

Author (s)	Publication year	Study location	Cases (N)	Study Period	Population-based	Adjustment[A]	Non-syndromic[B]
Morera et al.	2006	France	225	2002-2004	No	No	No
Nelson et al.	2005	United States	9,124	1988-2000	No	Yes	No
Porter et al.	2005	Washington State	2,155	1987-1997	Yes	Yes	No
Sørensen et al.	2005	Denmark	319	1989-2002	Yes	Yes	No
Ahmed et al.	2004	Scotland	2, 816	1988–1997	Yes	Yes	No
Aschim et al.	2004	Norway	2,382	1967-1998	Yes	Yes	No
Pierik et al.	2004	Netherlands	56	1999- 2001	Yes	Yes	No
Reefhuis and Honein	2004	Atlanta	-[D]	1968-2000	Yes	Yes	Yes
Skriver et al.	2004	Denmark	3,242	1983-2002	Yes	No	No
Aho et al.	2003	Finland	1,536	1970-1986	Yes	No	No
Carmichael et al.	2003	California	5,838	1984-1997	Yes	Yes	Yes
Fredell et al.	2002	Sweden	1,722	1970-1997	No	No	No
Hussain et al.	2002	Connecticut	112	1987-2000	No	No	Yes
Kallen	2002	Sweden	3,262	1983-1996	Yes	Yes	Yes
Fisch et al.	2001	New York and California	-[D]	1983-1996	Yes	No	No
North et al.	2000	England	51	1991-1992	Yes	Yes	No
Akre et al.	1999	Sweden	1,220	1983-1993	Yes	Yes	No
Weidner et al.	1999	Denmark	1,345	1983-1992	Yes	Yes	No
McIntosh et al.	1995	British Columbia	933	1952-1973	Yes	Yes	No
Stoll et al.	1990	France	176	1979-1987	No	No	No
Calzolari et al.	1986	Italy	168	1978-1983	No	No	No
Roberts and Lloyd	1973	Wales	93	1964-1966	Yes	No	No
Wehrung and Hay	1970	United States	5,145	1962-1965	Yes	No	No

[A] Adjusted effect measures reported.
[B] Analyses of non-syndromic or isolated hypospadias.
[C] National Birth Defects Prevention Study.
[D] Not specified.

When patients at a hospital or clinic are ascertained for a study, it stands to reason that the only potential study subjects would be those that sought healthcare at that facility. There might be non-random reasons why someone would not go to a particular healthcare facility, for example, the cost of medical care or the distance to travel to that facility might preclude an individual from accessing healthcare there. Therefore, the study might be biased in that the only potential participants would be those that can either afford to seek medical care at, or that live in relative proximity to, the facility. Furthermore, these individuals might be different from those who did not seek medical care at that facility (or elsewhere) and would thus bias the results obtained from that dataset.

Additionally, if the study design requires informed consent of the study subjects prior to obtaining data (as opposed to accessing de-identified medical record or registry data), this may introduce another level of selection bias, as eligible participants may or may not elect to participate based on a known or unknown modifier. In effect, those that consent to participation may, in some way, be different from those that reject participation, and possibly bias the results obtained from the dataset.

This issue with selection bias is greatly minimized in population-based studies, in which individuals are sampled from the general population or every eligible individual in the general population is included. The majority of the studies on hypospadias (Table 1) are population-based, where data is obtained from birth defect registries (Agopian et al., 2014; Carmichael et al., 2003; Marengo et al., 2013; Meyer et al., 2006; Reefhuis and Honein, 2004), vital statistic records (e.g., birth certificates) (Porter et al., 2005; Sorensen et al., 2005), national healthcare registries (Aho et al., 2003; Jin et al., 2010; Nelson et al., 2005) or from multiple registries (Ahmed et al., 2004; Kallen, 2002; Mavrogenis et al., 2014). Furthermore, when everyone in the population is ascertained, these studies are optimal sources for information regarding the prevalence of hypospadias in those specific regions or populations.

Case Definitions

Once a data source has been selected, it is imperative to have a clear definition of what constitutes a case (or a control, if applicable). Nearly all the studies on hypospadias have clearly stated case definitions based on standardized codes for birth defects (e.g., ICD-9, BPA, or EUROCAT). Some also stratify the results based on the morphology and meatal location of the defect (first-, second-, or third-degree). This is important, as the phenotypic variability in hypospadias may be due to heterogeneity in the etiology (van Rooij et al., 2013).

Although information on the penile phenotype is usually provided, few reports have offered information on or attempt to stratify by the presence or absence of other birth defects. Isolated cases of hypospadias are those in which the penile defect occurs in the absence of any other major congenital malformation or anomaly. A non-isolated defect occurs in the presence of one or more additional major congenital anomalies in the child. It is possible that the etiology (environmental or genetic) of isolated and non-isolated defects may be different. For example, the genetic polymorphism or mutation that might give rise to an isolated defect may be different from one that results in multiple defects.

Therefore, when describing exposures associated with hypospadias, it is possible that including all defects into the same diagnostic category may result in a heterogeneous group of cases. This heterogeneous group may fail to yield a significant association with an exposure that is associated with a specific type of hypospadias. Therefore, it is suggested that more homogeneous groups (e.g., isolated hypospadias) be analyzed when possible. Many studies do not state whether non-isolated cases are included or excluded in the analysis, though some explicitly state either that non-isolated cases were excluded from analysis or analyzed separately from the isolated cases (Abdullah et al., 2007a; Abdullah et al., 2007b; Aberg et al., 2001; Agopian et al., 2014; Carmichael et al., 2003; Hussain et al., 2002; Kallen, 2002; Mavrogenis et al., 2014).

Furthermore, there is a subset of non-isolated cases in which the birth defects present are due to an underlying genetic syndrome or chromosome abnormality, and these are referred to as syndromic cases. Because the etiology of hypospadias in these individuals is expected to be different than those with non-syndromic hypospadias, syndromic cases should be excluded from analyses; however, many reports do not specify how cases with syndromes were dealt with.

Some studies have evaluated a broader group of male genital defects overall, or all urogenital defects, regardless of sex, rather than hypospadias specifically. Because this may represent a very heterogeneous group with respect to etiology, it may be difficult to interpret results from such studies.

Due to all these considerations, a reviewer of literature should be cognizant of the inclusion or exclusion of non-isolated/syndromic cases in the analysis.

Sample Size

Epidemiological studies attempt to provide an estimate of the true relationship between characteristics and outcomes in a population, for example, an estimate of maternal exposure to a teratogen and risk for hypospadias in offspring. However, it is often not feasible to collect data on every individual in the population. Instead, investigators collect a "sample" of male children and query the relevant information only from then.

This "sampling" gives rise to "sampling error", since the results from a study are dependent on who is selected for participation in the study. If two investigators separately and randomly sample 100 individuals from a total population of 10,000, it is very unlikely that they will select the exact same 100 individuals. There might be a few sampled into both studies, but the majority of the individuals will probably be different between the studies. Therefore, the results from the two studies may be different depending on who participated in which study. Furthermore, since only a small subset of individuals from the whole population were selected for the study, it is possible that the estimate obtained in the study is different from the true value of the population parameter being measured. The randomness of who participates in a study (the chance of inclusion into the study) and the sampling error that stems from it is present in most studies.

One way to reduce this error is to increase the number of individuals being sampled into the study (i.e., increase the "sample size"). In the above example, if each investigator was sampling 2,000 individuals out of the 10,000, then the sample would include a much larger proportion of all individuals present in the study. This means that the estimate calculated in the sample will more closely approximate the true population parameter. Furthermore, since samples taken by different investigators will each have a greater proportion of the population, the likelihood of the same individual being in both studies will be much higher. This in turn will cause the two study estimates to be more similar to each other.

Therefore, the increase in sample size results in a more precise estimate of the truth, i.e., it has more statistical "power." Specifically, power refers to the probability of detecting a significant association when one exists. Conversely, a study with a low sample size will have a greater degree of variability in the point estimate, and thus low power. Even if every subject in the small population is analyzed, the study may have insufficient power to detect modest associations. Since sample size influences the precision of the estimate, it is important to recognize the number of participants in studies being compared.

In epidemiologic studies of hypospadias, the sample size ranges considerably, for example, from 34 cases in a clinic-based retrospective case-control study (Akin et al., 2011) to 16,813 cases from a large population-based birth defects registry (Agopian et al., 2014). In summary, results from larger samples should often be considered with a stronger weight that those from small samples.

Type of Statistic Reported

Another factor to consider when comparing and contrasting studies is the type of statistic described. Some studies report only absolute estimates of risk (e.g., overall birth prevalence), which are of limited use for identifying hypospadias risk factors. It is more helpful when studies report relative estimates of risk (e.g., odds ratios), which allow for comparisons between a group of interested (e.g., exposed) and a reference (e.g., unexposed) comparison group.

Some studies report p-values rather than point estimates (e.g., odds ratios). While p-values can indicate statistically significant differences, without a reported point estimate, there is no indication of the direction or magnitude of the effect from a p-value. Further, 95% confidence intervals (CIs) provide more information than p-values about the precision of an effect, as 95% CIs indicate the range over which the true point estimate is expected to fall.

Accounting for Confounding

Not all studies account for potential confounders. Confounding occurs when the relationship observed between two variables is distorted by a third variable. Although most studies do adjust for confounding, some do not (Table 1). Lack of adjustment for confounding is often driven by the study design. Relying on previously collected data means that the investigator would not be able to assess confounding if data on the variable of interest is lacking. Even if the data were available, a small sample size might preclude the ability to perform any meaningful adjusted analysis, because adjusting for confounders (i.e., adding additional variables in the statistical model) reduces power. As mentioned previously, an adequate sample size is critical for obtaining precise estimates of a population parameter. If the data is adjusted on one or more variables, the total sample size will be "spread out" between the various strata.

The resultant small sample sizes within each strata might then lead to underpowered comparisons between the strata. This may result in a lack of significant associations in a moderate-sized study that adjusts for many variables.

Summary

When considering the descriptive epidemiology of hypospadias, it is important to consider the limitations and strengths of various study designs, sampling techniques, and statistical analyses. Also, when multiple studies have been performed, it is important to assess each study not only on its own but also as part of the larger body of literature on the topic. Consistency of the direction and magnitude of point estimates (e.g., odds ratios) across studies, even without statistical significance in all of them, should provide confidence in assuming that the estimated trends are a true reflection of effects. Conversely, effects from studies which have not been replicated, especially those with small sample sizes, should provide pause for consideration of potential biases and errors. The following sections will attempt to summarize the main findings from the literature published on hypospadias over the last few decades in light of strengths and limitations of the studies.

Temporal Trends

In past decades, there has been concern about the possibility that the prevalence of hypospadias has increased. Several older studies suggested that the prevalence was increasing in several European countries as well as in the U.S. during the period between the late 1960s and early 1990s (Bjerkedal and Bakketeig, 1975; Czeizel, 1985; International Clearinghouse for Birth Defects Monitoring Systems, 1991; Kallen et al., 1986; Kallen and Winberg, 1979; 1982; Matlai and Beral, 1985; Paulozzi et al., 1997). Initially, it was proposed that this increase might be partially explained by use of environmental endocrine disrupting chemicals. However, subsequent reports suggested that the prevalence had stabilized or was decreasing during the period between the mid-1980s to the present in many countries and regions studied (Abdullah et al., 2007a; Ahmed et al., 2004; Aho et al., 2000; Correa et al., 2007; Dolk et al., 2004; Elliott et al., 2011; Fisch et al., 2001; Ghirri et al., 2009; Kurahashi et al., 2004; Loane et al., 2011; Martinez-Frias et al., 2004; Paulozzi, 1999; Porter et al., 2005). Increases in the prevalence of hypospadias during this time period has occurred only in isolated areas and/or during specific time periods, and in these areas, changes in the way hypospadias is identified, reported, and/or ascertained are likely responsible for at least part of the observed prevalence increase (Canon et al., 2012; Carmichael et al., 2012; Nissen et al., 2014; Nordenvall et al., 2014).

Seasonal effects (i.e., associations with factors related to daylight, climate, or temperature) have been reported in some older studies (Angerpointner, 1984; Avellan, 1977; Czeizel et al., 1979; Kallen et al., 1986; Roberts and Lloyd, 1973; Svensson, 1979; Wehrung and Hay, 1970); however, more recent studies have not reported seasonal variation in hypospadias risk (Agopian et al., 2014; Calzolari et al., 1986; Castilla et al., 1990; Jin et al., 2010; Morera et al., 2006; Nazer et al., 1992; Skriver et al., 2004; Stoll et al., 1990).

Geographic Trends

There have been large differences in the reported prevalence of hypospadias between countries. As an extreme example, the birth prevalence of hypospadias in Finland during 1997-2004 was 0.27%, whereas the birth prevalence in Denmark during 1997-2004 was 1.03% (Boisen et al., 2005). A large part of these differences between registry systems is likely due to differences in ascertainment, reporting, and case definitions. For example, some systems do not include mild cases of hypospadias.

Geographic differences between different regions within the same reporting system have also been reported (Abdullah et al., 2007b; Agopian et al., 2014; Aviles et al., 2014; Canon et al., 2012; Pohl et al., 2007). In some instances, it has been suggested that these differences may be related to differences in exposure to environmental risk factors (Chul Kim et al., 2011; Winston et al., 2014); however, it is difficult to make definitive conclusions from these ecologic comparisons. Several studies have more thoroughly evaluated residential proximity to factors associated with environmental risk factors, though these studies are beyond the scope of this review. In one study, hypospadias risk was reported to increase with lower altitude (Castilla et al., 1990). It is possible that observed geographic differences, even within the same reporting system, are partially influenced by variation in ascertainment and reporting.

Most Established Associations

Family History

Most birth defects are considered to be complex traits, involving a combination of both genetic and non-genetic risk factors. Evidence for a genetic contribution to risk is apparent from patterns of occurrence of birth defects in family members, with a higher prevalence in relatives of a case compared to the general population. Associations between hypospadias risk and a history of hypospadias in a family member have been reported (Bauer et al., 1979; Brouwers et al., 2010; Calzolari et al., 1986; Fredell et al., 2002; Mohammadzadeh et al., 2011; Schnack et al., 2008; Stoll et al., 1990; van Rooij et al., 2013; Woud et al., 2014). Specifically, the risk of hypospadias to a brother of an affected case is 6-17% (Table 2) (Calzolari et al., 1986; Schnack et al., 2008; Stoll et al., 1990) and the heritability is estimated to be 57-67% (Calzolari et al., 1986; Stoll et al., 1990). A family history of hypospadias is the strongest known risk factor (odds ratio: 13-26) (Schnack et al., 2008; Woud et al., 2014); however, the majority of cases occur in individuals without a family history.

Table 2. Summary of effects of some of the most established hypospadias risk factors

Risk factor	Suspected odds ratio
History of hypospadias in a brother	6-17
Low parity	1.3-2
Multiple gestation pregnancy	1.5-3
Non-Hispanic white maternal race/ethnicity	1.2-3

The results from studies comparing risk related to family history by hypospadias severity have been mixed (Bauer et al., 1979; Brouwers et al., 2010; Fredell et al., 2002; van Rooij et al., 2013; Woud et al., 2014); however, the more recent studies suggest that family history is a stronger risk factor for less severe forms of hypospadias compared to more severe forms (e.g., second-degree versus third-degree). In one study, the risk for hypospadias in offspring was increased when there was a previous pregnancy with any congenital anomaly (Ahmed et al., 2004). Future research will identify specific genetic factors that influence hypospadias risk.

Parity

A number of studies have reported a higher risk of hypospadias among offspring of women with low parity (e.g., nulliparous) (Agopian et al., 2014; Akre et al., 1999; Aschim et al., 2004; Carmichael et al., 2007; Carmichael et al., 2003; Chen and Woolley, 1971; Czeizel et al., 1979; Hay and Barbano, 1972; Hussain et al., 2002; Jin et al., 2010; Kallen, 2002; Mavrogenis et al., 2014; Meyer et al., 2006; Morera et al., 2006; Nassar et al., 2010; North and Golding, 2000; Sorensen et al., 2005; van Rooij et al., 2013; Weidner et al., 1999; Woud et al., 2014). It has been proposed that this observed association may implicate the role of abnormal estrogen levels in the development of hypospadias, as women have been shown to have higher levels of estradiol in their first pregnancy compared to subsequent pregnancies (Storgaard et al., 2006).

Plurality

The relationship between multiple gestation pregnancies and birth defects can be complicated to evaluate because of the possibility that selection against severe phenotypes in twins (e.g., impaired placental function) may be higher than selection against the same phenotype in singletons (Kallen et al., 1986); however, this form of selection bias would most likely bias results towards a conclusion of no association between hypospadias and multiple gestation pregnancies. The majority of studies that have evaluated hypospadias risk among multiple gestation pregnancies have reported an increase in risk (Agopian et al., 2014; Akin et al., 2011; Akre et al., 1999; Aschim et al., 2004; Brouwers et al., 2007; Brouwers et al., 2010; Carmichael et al., 2007; Carmichael et al., 2003; Czeizel et al., 1979; Fredell et al., 2002; Funke et al., 2010; Jin et al., 2010; Kallen et al., 1986; Mastroiacovo et al., 1999; Mavrogenis et al., 2014; Morera et al., 2006; Nassar et al., 2010; Nordenvall et al., 2014; Roberts and Lloyd, 1973; Sun et al., 2009; van Rooij et al., 2013; Weidner et al., 1999; Woud et al., 2014). Most studies estimate that risk of hypospadias in a male in a multiple gestation pregnancy is 1.5-3 times higher than that in a singleton gestation pregnancy. It has been proposed that over-adjustment for birth weight may account for differences in reported effects among studies which estimated weaker magnitudes of association or non-significant results (van der Zanden et al., 2012). The available evidence suggests that risk is higher among male-male twin pairs (Ramos-Arroyo, 1991) and also higher among monozygotic twins (Czeizel et al., 1979; Fredell et al., 2002; Roberts and Lloyd, 1973). It has been hypothesized that the association between hypospadias and a multiple gestation pregnancy may support a developmental mechanism involving abnormal estrogen levels, as estriol levels are 2-3 times higher in twin pregnancies compared to singleton pregnancies from a few weeks after conception (Storgaard et al., 2006).

Race/Ethnicity

The risk of hypospadias is generally reported to be higher among offspring of non-Hispanic white and Asian/Pacific Islander women compared to other race ethnicities, with particularly low risk in Hispanics (Adams et al., 2011; Agopian et al., 2014; Canon et al., 2012; Carmichael et al., 2003; Chavez et al., 1988; Chung and Myrianthopoulos, 1968; Leck and Lancashire, 1995; Lowry et al., 1986; Nassar et al., 2010; Nelson et al., 2005; Nordenvall et al., 2014; Pohl et al., 2007; Porter et al., 2005; Winston et al., 2014; Woud et al., 2014).

By contrast, for third-degree hypospadias, Woud et al. reported the highest hypospadias risk among offspring of Asian/Pacific Islander women followed by non-Hispanic black women and similar risk among other race/ethnicities (Woud et al., 2014). However, for third-degree hypospadias, Canon et al. reported similar risk in offspring of non-Hispanic white and black women and lower risk in offspring of Hispanic women and women of other/unknown race/ethnicities (Canon et al., 2012). Compared to non-Hispanic white women, the risk of hypospadias among births to Vietnamese women in California was lower (Shaw et al., 2002) and the risk among births to Japanese women in Hawaii was lower (Forrester and Merz, 2006). It is unclear if differences in race/ethnicity reflect genetic differences versus differences in non-genetic factors (e.g., diet, behavior differences, socio-economic factors).

Differences in results between studies may be in part due to differences in the racial/ethnic distribution between populations and subsequent differences in how racial/ethnic categories were characterized (e.g., black versus non-Hispanic black) and how comparisons were conducted (e.g., non-Hispanic white compared to non-Hispanic black versus non-Hispanic white compared to other race/ethnicities).

Suspected Associations

Education

Several studies, many of which were conducted in the United States have reported the risk of hypospadias to be higher among offspring of women with a higher level of education (Adams et al., 2011; Agopian et al., 2014; Berkowitz et al., 1995; Carmichael et al., 2007; Carmichael et al., 2003; Christensen et al., 2013; Jin et al., 2010; Winston et al., 2014; Woud et al., 2014). However, some studies did not report this association (Akre et al., 2008; Giordano et al., 2010) and some studies have reported a higher risk of hypospadias among offspring of women with lower levels of education (Brouwers et al., 2007; Carbone et al., 2007; Kallen, 2002; Pierik et al., 2004), though all of these studies were conducted in Europe, which suggests that there may be differences between the effect of maternal education between countries.

Socioeconomic Status

Socioeconomic status involves a variety of different factors, and only a limited number of studies have evaluated the relationship between such factors and hypospadias. The limited available evidence suggests that several factors that are generally thought to represent higher socioeconomic status may be associated with hypospadias, though it is not clear what mechanisms may be involved. For example, women with a higher household income have been shown to have a higher risk for hypospadias in one study (Nelson et al., 2005). In Puerto Rico, risk for hypospadias was higher among offspring of women with private health insurance compared to government health insurance (Aviles et al., 2014). Similarly, the risk among women with private/HMO/Medicare coverage was higher compared to women with Medicaid/other/no coverage (Nelson et al., 2005). However, factors representing lower socioeconomic status have also been associated with hypospadias. In Scotland, the highest risk of hypospadias was reported in areas that had Carstairs deprivation scores representing the least deprived areas (Ahmed et al., 2004). By contrast, risk for hypospadias did not vary by percentage of inhabitants in the highest or lowest social class in Finland (Aho et al., 2003).

Further study of factors that represent socioeconomic status is needed to better understand the dynamics involved, especially the evaluation of individual-level variables (with appropriate adjustment for potential confounders). The reported associations between hypospadias and factors related to higher socioeconomic status seem consistent with reported associations between hypospadias and non-Hispanic white race/ethnicity and higher level of maternal education.

Age

While the majority of studies have not reported an association between maternal or paternal age and risk of hypospadias in offspring (Agopian et al., 2014; Akre et al., 1999; Aschim et al., 2004; Brouwers et al., 2007, Calzolari et al., 1986; Carbone et al., 2007; Chambers and Malone, 1999; Czeizel et al., 1979; Ghirri et al., 2009; Hussain et al., 2002; Kallen and Winberg, 1982; Kallen, 2002; Lund et al., 2009; Materna-Kiryluk et al., 2009; Meyer et al., 2006; Morera et al., 2006; Nassar et al., 2010; Sorensen et al., 2005; Stoll et al., 1990; Sun et al., 2009; Weidner et al., 1999), numerous studies have reported an association with higher maternal age (Ahmed et al., 2004; Akin et al., 2011; Carmichael et al., 2007; Carmichael et al., 2003; Fisch et al., 2001; Fisch et al., 2009; Hussain et al., 2002; Porter et al., 2005; Reefhuis and Honein, 2004; Winston et al., 2014; Woud et al., 2014) or lower or higher paternal age (Materna-Kiryluk et al., 2009; Mavrogenis et al., 2014; McIntosh et al., 1995). Differences in results may be related to differences in categorizing age (e.g., continuous versus categorical) or modeling (e.g., differences in co-variables).

Body Mass Index

High, as compared to normal, body mass index appears to be a strong risk factor for a variety of birth defects. Because having a high body mass index (i.e., being overweight or obese) is a common exposure, it is a very important potential risk factor to consider for birth defects. Multiple studies have reported on associations between maternal obesity or overweight status and hypospadias in offspring (Akre et al., 2008; Blomberg and Kallen, 2010; Carmichael et al., 2007; Giordano et al., 2010; Marengo et al., 2013; Nordenvall et al., 2014; van Rooij et al., 2013; Waller et al., 2007). Carmichael et al. reported a particularly elevated risk (odds ratio: 12.5, 95% confidence interval: 5.1-30.8) among women who were primiparous, age ≥35 years, and had a body mass index of >26 compared to those who were multiparous, age <30 years and had a body mass index of ≤26 (Carmichael et al., 2007).

Another study did not find an association between overweight or obese status and hypospadias, but did find an association between underweight versus normal weight status and hypospadias (Rankin et al., 2010). Other studies have not reported an association between hypospadias and maternal body mass index (Adams et al., 2011; Christensen et al., 2013; Woud et al., 2014).

Differences in the way that studies have categorized and compared body mass index (e.g., obese versus non-obese as compared to normal weight versus overweight or obese) may explain some of the differences in results between studies. As endogenous levels of free estradiol during pregnancy increase with increasing maternal body mass index, the association between maternal body mass index and hypospadias may provide further evidence supporting the role of a mechanism involving endocrine disruption.

Maternal Diabetes

Whereas a number of birth defects have been associated with maternal diabetes, only a few studies have reported associations between pre-gestational diabetes and hypospadias, but not gestational diabetes and hypospadias (Aberg et al., 2001; Porter et al., 2005). In another study, gestational diabetes was associated with hypospadias (Mavrogenis et al., 2014).

A study from the National Birth Defects Prevention Study reported strong, statistically significant associations between non-isolated hypospadias (i.e., hypospadias present with additional birth defects) and both pre-gestational and gestational diabetes (Correa et al., 2008a) and another analysis from the same data source reported similar associations with pre-gestational diabetes and hypospadias, but not gestational diabetes (Woud et al., 2014). Other studies have not reported on an association between diabetes and hypospadias (Agopian et al., 2014; Aschim et al., 2004; Becerra et al., 1990; Brouwers et al., 2010; Hussain et al., 2002; Kallen, 1988; Morera et al., 2006; Polednak and Janerich, 1983; Ramos-Arroyo et al., 1992; Sorensen et al., 2005; Stoll et al., 1990; Sun et al., 2009; Trabert et al., 2014; Winston et al., 2014). A number of these studies had small sample sizes, which makes it difficult to draw definitive conclusions from their results, and many of these studies reported a moderate-to-strong positive magnitude of effect, albeit non-significant. Evaluating maternal diabetes and risk for hypospadias can be challenging, as existing sources of data (e.g., vital records) may have incomplete information on maternal diabetes, which could potentially introduce selection bias.

Some data sources may not distinguish between gestational versus pre-gestational diabetes, which could have different effects on hypospadias risk. Further, because gestational and pre-gestational diabetes are relatively rare during pregnancy, very large samples are required for sufficient power to detect statistically significant associations. Given the mixed results and limitations of many of the studies reporting null results, further study of the relationship between hypospadias and maternal diabetes is indicated.

Assisted Reproductive Technology

Several studies have reported a higher risk for hypospadias among pregnancies that have used reproductive fertility treatments or assisted reproductive technologies (Brouwers et al., 2007; Brouwers et al., 2010; Carmichael et al., 2007; Silver et al., 1999), including intra-cytoplasmic sperm injection (Bang et al., 2013; Ericson and Kallen, 2001; Fedder et al., 2007; Funke et al., 2010; Kallen et al., 2005; Nordenvall et al., 2014; Pinborg et al., 2004; Wennerholm et al., 2000). However, in vitro fertilization was not reported to be associated with hypospadias in a number of studies (Bonduelle et al., 1995; Ericson and Kallen, 2001; Funke et al., 2010; Hansen et al., 2002; Kallen et al., 2010; Morera et al., 2006; Oldereid et al., 2003), although results from some of these studies were inconclusive. As assisted reproductive technologies often involve hormonal stimulation, the reported associations may further support a role of endocrine disruption on hypospadias risk. However, it is difficult to determine whether any potential increase in risk is due to the fertility procedure versus an underlying condition (i.e., confounding by indication).

Maternal Hypertension and Pre-Eclampsia

An association between maternal hypertension during pregnancy and increased risk for hypospadias has been reported in several studies (Adams et al., 2011; Akre et al., 2008; Aschim et al., 2004; Brouwers et al., 2010; Caton et al., 2008; Morera et al., 2006; Sun et al., 2009; van der Zanden et al., 2012; van Rooij et al., 2013; Woud et al., 2014). Similar associations have been reported between hypospadias and maternal pre-eclampsia (Adams et al., 2011; Akre et al., 1999; Aschim et al., 2004; Brouwers et al., 2010; Morera et al., 2006; Sorensen et al., 2005; Sun et al., 2009). Both of these maternal conditions are suspected to be associated with placental dysfunction and may compromise uteroplacental perfusion (Caton et al., 2008). It is challenging to separate the potential effects of the underlying hypertension versus effects of hypertension medications.

Other Parental Factors

Several other associations have been reported. Maternal thyroid disease has been associated with hypospadias in one study (Browne et al., 2009). A younger maternal age at menarche has been associated with hypospadias risk in some (Calzolari et al., 1986; Giordano et al., 2010; Morera et al., 2006) but not all (Akre et al., 2008; Stoll et al., 1990) studies that have evaluated the association. Poor self-reported general health was associated with hypospadias as compared to good general health (Pierik et al., 2004). The risk of hypospadias has also been reported to be higher among offspring of women without early prenatal care (Meyer et al., 2006). Other maternal behaviors (e.g., smoking, use of folic acid) have also been studied, but are beyond the scope of this review.

Potential Mechanisms Implicated

The observed associations from descriptive epidemiologic studies can be helpful in identifying potential pathways and mechanisms that may be involved in the development of hypospadias. A variety of descriptive factors that have been associated with hypospadias in epidemiologic studies (e.g., low parity, multiple gestation pregnancy, high body mass index, fertility-related procedures, age at menarche, thyroid disease) support the idea that endocrine disruption may be involved in the etiology of hypospadias in some instances. The potential role of endocrine disrupting chemicals in the environment has also been studied, but remains unclear.

Some factors that tend to be correlated with higher socioeconomic status (e.g., non-Hispanic white race/ethnicity, higher education, higher household income, private insurance) have been reported to be associated with hypospadias. These associations suggest a pattern that is uncommon compared to many other birth defects that are associated with variables correlated with lower socioeconomic status. The notion that hypospadias is associated with factors related to higher socioeconomic status is somewhat enigmatic, considering that many of these women likely have better access to health resources and nutrition and are more likely to use folic acid and avoid unhealthy behaviors during pregnancy, such as drinking alcohol or smoking. More research in this area is needed to identify more specific risk factors related to higher socioeconomic status that are associated with hypospadias and then to elucidate the mechanisms involved.

Etiologic Heterogeneity

It is unclear if the etiology of more severe forms of hypospadias (e.g., third-degree) are distinct from less severe forms (e.g., second-degree). Similarly, it is unclearl if isolated hypospadias (i.e., no other birth defects present) is etiologically distinct from non-syndromic hypospadias in the presence of additional non-genital birth defects. A limited number of studies have evaluated differences in the descriptive epidemiology of hypospadias subgroups, based on degree of severity (Agopian et al., 2014; Canon et al., 2012; Woud et al., 2014) or isolated versus non-isolated status (Correa et al., 2008b).

The results from these studies suggest that there are both similarities and differences in the effects of different suspected risk factors. In other words, these findings support the notion that there are etiologic similarities between hypospadias subgroups, but that there may also be mechanisms that are distinct to particular phenotypic subgroups. Therefore, it is likely that some differences between the observed results among studies that have not considered the etiologic heterogeneity in hypospadias may be related to differences in case definitions (e.g., second-degree versus degree unspecified; isolated hypospadias versus hypospadias without regard to additional defects).

Along the same lines, some similar epidemiologic trends have been reported between hypospadias and other male genital defects, such as cryptorchidism (Adams et al., 2011; Agopian et al., 2014; Akre et al., 1999; Carbone et al., 2007; Pierik et al., 2004; Weidner et al., 1999). These findings suggest that the broader group of male genital defects may represent a spectrum of inter-related defects to a certain extent. More research is needed to better understand the potential overlap between hypospadias and related phenotypes.

Future Directions

Birth defects surveillance systems and epidemiologic researchers should strive to better calibrate hypospadias case definitions and ascertainment approaches, in order to more completely capture the prevalence of these conditions and reduce the potential for selection bias and artifactual differences between surveillance systems. Because very large numbers are required to study hypospadias, especially when evaluating rare exposures, expanded collection approaches would be helpful. As many of the existing data sources are limited to information available from vital records, efforts to collect data on novel characteristics and exposures will be critical for the future. Thoughtful epidemiologic analyses, considering the potential etiologic heterogeneity within hypospadias phenotypes and accounting for potential sources of bias, will also be of paramount importance.

Conclusion

Several studies have assessed the descriptive epidemiology of hypospadias and identified a risk profile that has provided clues about etiologic mechanisms involved. These mechanisms should be further evaluated in more targeted analytic epidemiologic studies. Further research is needed to confirm or refute the inconsistent associations that have been observed and to identify associations with characteristics that have not yet been evaluated.

References

Abdullah NA, Pearce MS, Parker L, Wilkinson JR, Jaffray B, McNally RJ. 2007a. Birth prevalence of cryptorchidism and hypospadias in northern England, 1993-2000. *Arch. Dis. Child* 92:576-579.

Abdullah NA, Pearce MS, Parker L, Wilkinson JR, McNally RJ. 2007b. Evidence of an environmental contribution to the aetiology of cryptorchidism and hypospadias? *Eur. J. Epidemiol.* 22:615-620.

Aberg A, Westbom L, Kallen B. 2001. Congenital malformations among infants whose mothers had gestational diabetes or preexisting diabetes. *Early Hum. Dev* .61:85-95.

Adams SV, Hastert TA, Huang Y, Starr JR. 2011. No association between maternal pre-pregnancy obesity and risk of hypospadias or cryptorchidism in male newborns. *Birt Defects Res. A. Clin. Mol. Teratol.* 91:241-248.

Agopian AJ, Langlois PH, Ramakrishnan A, Canfield MA. 2014. Epidemiologic features of male genital malformations and subtypes in Texas. *Am. J. Med. Genet. A* 164A:943-949.

Ahmed SF, Dobbie R, Finlayson AR, Gilbert J, Youngson G, Chalmers J, Stone D. 2004. Prevalence of hypospadias and other genital anomalies among singleton births, 1988-1997, in Scotland. *Arch. Dis. Child Fetal Neonatal Ed* 89:F149-151.

Aho M, Koivisto AM, Tammela TL, Auvinen A. 2000. Is the incidence of hypospadias increasing? Analysis of Finnish hospital discharge data 1970-1994. *Environ. Health Perspect* 108:463-465.

Aho MO, Koivisto AM, Tammela TL, Auvinen AP. 2003. Geographical differences in the prevalence of hypospadias in Finland. *Environ. Res.* 92:118-123.

Akin Y, Ercan O, Telatar B, Tarhan F, Comert S. 2011. Hypospadias in Istanbul: incidence and risk factors. *Pediatr Int.* 53:754-760.

Akre O, Boyd HA, Ahlgren M, Wilbrand K, Westergaard T, Hjalgrim H, Nordenskjold A, Ekbom A, Melbye M. 2008. Maternal and gestational risk factors for hypospadias. *Environ. Health Perspect* 116:1071-1076.

Akre O, Lipworth L, Cnattingius S, Sparen P, Ekbom A. 1999. Risk factor patterns for cryptorchidism and hypospadias. *Epidemiology* 10:364-369.

Angerpointner TA. 1984. Hypospadias--genetics, epidemiology and other possible aetiological influences. *Z Kinderchir* 39:112-118.

Aschim EL, Haugen TB, Tretli S, Daltveit AK, Grotmol T. 2004. Risk factors for hypospadias in Norwegian boys - association with testicular dysgenesis syndrome? *Int. J. Androl.* 27:213-221.

Avellan L. 1977. On aetiological factors in hypospadias. *Scand. J. Plast. Reconstr Surg.* 11:115-123.

Aviles LA, Alvelo-Maldonado L, Padro-Mojica I, Seguinot J, Jorge JC. 2014. Risk factors, prevalence trend, and clustering of hypospadias cases in Puerto Rico. *J. Pediatr Urol.*

Bang JK, Lyu SW, Choi J, Lee DR, Yoon TK, Song SH. 2013. Does infertility treatment increase male reproductive tract disorder? *Urology* 81:644-648.

Bauer SB, Bull MJ, Retik AB. 1979. Hypospadias: a familial study. *J. Urol.* 121:474-477.

Becerra JE, Khoury MJ, Cordero JF, Erickson JD. 1990. Diabetes mellitus during pregnancy and the risks for specific birth defects: a population-based case-control study. *Pediatrics* 85:1-9.

Berkowitz GS, Lapinski RH, Godbold JH, Dolgin SE, Holzman IR. 1995. Maternal and neonatal risk factors for cryptorchidism. *Epidemiology* 6:127-131.

Bjerkedal T, Bakketeig LS. 1975. Surveillance of congenital malformations and other conditions of the newborn. *Int. J. Epidemiol.* 4:31-36.

Blomberg MI, Kallen B. 2010. Maternal obesity and morbid obesity: the risk for birth defects in the offspring. *Birt Defects Res. A. Clin. Mol. Teratol.* 88:35-40.

Boisen KA, Chellakooty M, Schmidt IM, Kai CM, Damgaard IN, Suomi AM, Toppari J, Skakkebaek NE, Main KM. 2005. Hypospadias in a cohort of 1072 Danish newborn boys: prevalence and relationship to placental weight, anthropometrical measurements at birth, and reproductive hormone levels at three months of age. *J. Clin. Endocrinol. Metab.* 90:4041-4046.

Bonduelle M, Legein J, Derde MP, Buysse A, Schietecatte J, Wisanto A, Devroey P, Van Steirteghem A, Liebaers I. 1995. Comparative follow-up study of 130 children born after intracytoplasmic sperm injection and 130 children born after in-vitro fertilization. *Hum. Reprod.* 10:3327-3331.

Brouwers MM, Feitz WF, Roelofs LA, Kiemeney LA, de Gier RP, Roeleveld N. 2007. Risk factors for hypospadias. *Eur. J. Pediatr* 166:671-678.

Brouwers MM, van der Zanden LF, de Gier RP, Barten EJ, Zielhuis GA, Feitz WF, Roeleveld N. 2010. Hypospadias: risk factor patterns and different phenotypes. *BJU Int. 105*:254-262.

Browne ML, Rasmussen SA, Hoyt AT, Waller DK, Druschel CM, Caton AR, Canfield MA, Lin AE, Carmichael SL, Romitti PA. 2009. Maternal thyroid disease, thyroid medication use, and selected birth defects in the National Birth Defects Prevention Study. *Birt Defects Res. A. Clin. Mol. Teratol.* 85:621-628.

Calzolari E, Contiero MR, Roncarati E, Mattiuz PL, Volpato S. 1986. Aetiological factors in hypospadias. *J. Med. Genet.* 23:333-337.

Canon S, Mosley B, Chipollini J, Purifoy JA, Hobbs C. 2012. Epidemiological assessment of hypospadias by degree of severity. *J. Urol.* 188:2362-2366.

Carbone P, Giordano F, Nori F, Mantovani A, Taruscio D, Lauria L, Figa-Talamanca I. 2007. The possible role of endocrine disrupting chemicals in the aetiology of cryptorchidism and hypospadias: a population-based case-control study in rural Sicily. *Int. J. Androl.* 30:3-13.

Carlson WH, Kisely SR, MacLellan DL. 2009. Maternal and fetal risk factors associated with severity of hypospadias: a comparison of mild and severe cases. *J. Pediatr. Urol.* 5:283-286.

Carmichael SL, Shaw GM, Lammer EJ. 2012. Environmental and genetic contributors to hypospadias: A review of the epidemiologic evidence. *Birt Defects Res. A. Clin. Mol. Teratol.* 94:499-510.

Carmichael SL, Shaw GM, Laurent C, Olney RS, Lammer EJ. 2007. Maternal reproductive and demographic characteristics as risk factors for hypospadias. *Paediatr Perinat Epidemiol.* 21:210-218.

Carmichael SL, Shaw GM, Nelson V, Selvin S, Torfs CP, Curry CJ. 2003. Hypospadias in California: trends and descriptive epidemiology. *Epidemiology* 14:701-706.

Castilla EE, Orioli IM, Lugarinho R, Dutra GP, Lopez-Camelo JS, Campana HE, Spagnolo A, Mastroiacovo P. 1990. Monthly and seasonal variations in the frequency of congenital anomalies. *Int. J. Epidemiol.* 19:399-404.

Caton AR, Bell EM, Druschel CM, Werler MM, Mitchell AA, Browne ML, McNutt LA, Romitti PA, Olney RS, Correa A. 2008. Maternal hypertension, antihypertensive medication use, and the risk of severe hypospadias. *Birt Defects Res. A. Clin. Mol. Teratol.* 82:34-40.

Centers for Disease Control and Prevention. 1995. Economic costs of birth defects and cerebral palsy--United States, 1992. *MMWR Morbidity and mortality weekly report* 44:694-699.

Chambers EL, Malone PS. 1999. The incidence of hypospadias in two English cities: a case-control comparison of possible causal factors. *BJU Int.* 84:95-98.

Chavez GF, Cordero JF, Becerra JE. 1988. Leading major congenital malformations among minority groups in the United States, 1981-1986. MMWR CDC Surveill Summ 37:17-24.

Chen YC, Woolley PV, Jr. 1971. Genetic studies on hypospadias in males. *J. Med. Genet.* 8:153-159.

Christensen JS, Asklund C, Skakkebaek NE, Jorgensen N, Andersen HR, Jorgensen TM, Olsen LH, Hoyer AP, Moesgaard J, Thorup J, Jensen TK. 2013. Association between organic dietary choice during pregnancy and hypospadias in offspring: a study of mothers of 306 boys operated on for hypospadias. *J. Urol.* 189:1077-1082.

Christianson A, Howson CP, Modell B. 2006. March of Dimes Global Report on Birth Defects. White Plains, New York: March of Dimes Research Foundation. 1-76 p.

Chul Kim S, Kyoung Kwon S, Pyo Hong Y. 2011. Trends in the incidence of cryptorchidism and hypospadias of registry-based data in Korea: a comparison between industrialized areas of petrochemical estates and a non-industrialized area. *Asian J. Androl.* 13:715-718.

Chung CS, Myrianthopoulos NC. 1968. Racial and prenatal factors in major congenital malformations. *Am. J. Hum. Genet.* 20:44-60.

Correa A, Cragan JD, Kucik JE, Alverson CJ, Gilboa SM, Balakrishnan R, Strickland MJ, Duke CW, O'Leary LA, Riehle-Colarusso T, Siffel C, Gambrell D, Thompson D, Atkinson M, Chitra J. 2007. Reporting birth defects surveillance data 1968-2003. *Birt Defects Res. A. Clin. Mol. Teratol.* 79:65-186.

Correa A, Gilboa SM, Besser LM, Botto LD, Moore CA, Hobbs CA, Cleves MA, Riehle-Colarusso TJ, Waller DK, Reece EA. 2008a. Diabetes mellitus and birth defects. *Am. J. Obstet. Gynecol.* 199:237 e231-239.

Correa A, Gilboa SM, Besser LM, Botto LD, Moore CA, Hobbs CA, Cleves MA, Riehle-Colarusso TJ, Waller DK, Reece EA. 2008b. Diabetes mellitus and birth defects. *Am. J. Obstet. Gynecol.* 199:237 e231-239.

Czeizel A. 1985. Increasing trends in congenital malformations of male external genitalia. *Lancet* 1:462-463.

Czeizel A, Toth J, Erodi E. 1979. Aetiological studies of hypospadias in Hungary. *Hum. Hered* 29:166-171.

Dolk H, Vrijheid M, Scott JE, Addor MC, Botting B, de Vigan C, de Walle H, Garne E, Loane M, Pierini A, Garcia-Minaur S, Physick N, Tenconi R, Wiesel A, Calzolari E, Stone D. 2004. Toward the effective surveillance of hypospadias. *Environ. Health Perspect* 112:398-402.

Elliott CS, Halpern MS, Paik J, Maldonado Y, Shortliffe LD. 2011. Epidemiologic trends in penile anomalies and hypospadias in the state of California, 1985-2006. *J. Pediatr. Urol.* 7:294-298.

Elwood M. 2007. Critical Appraisal of Epidemiological Studies and Clinical Trials. third Ed. Oxford: Oxford University Press.

Ericson A, Kallen B. 2001. Congenital malformations in infants born after IVF: a population-based study. *Hum. Reprod.* 16:504-509.

Fedder J, Gabrielsen A, Humaidan P, Erb K, Ernst E, Loft A. 2007. Malformation rate and sex ratio in 412 children conceived with epididymal or testicular sperm. *Hum. Reprod.* 22:1080-1085.

Fisch H, Golden RJ, Libersen GL, Hyun GS, Madsen P, New MI, Hensle TW. 2001. Maternal age as a risk factor for hypospadias. *J. Urol.* 165:934-936.

Fisch H, Lambert SM, Hensle TW, Hyun G. 2009. Hypospadias rates in new york state are not increasing. *J. Urol.* 181:2291-2294.

Forrester MB, Merz RD. 2006. Rates for specific birth defects among offspring of Japanese mothers, Hawaii, 1986-2002. *Congenit Anom. (Kyoto)* 46:76-80.

Fredell L, Kockum I, Hansson E, Holmner S, Lundquist L, Lackgren G, Pedersen J, Stenberg A, Westbacke G, Nordenskjold A. 2002. Heredity of hypospadias and the significance of low birth weight. *J. Urol.* 167:1423-1427.

Funke S, Flach E, Kiss I, Sandor J, Vida G, Bodis J, Ertl T. 2010. Male reproductive tract abnormalities: more common after assisted reproduction? *Early Hum. Dev.* 86:547-550.

Ghirri P, Scaramuzzo RT, Bertelloni S, Pardi D, Celandroni A, Cocchi G, Danieli R, De Santis L, Di Stefano MC, Gerola O, Giuffre M, Gragnani GS, Magnani C, Meossi C, Merusi I, Sabatino G, Tumini S, Corsello G, Boldrini A. 2009. Prevalence of hypospadias in Italy according to severity, gestational age and birthweight: an epidemiological study. *Ital. J. Pediatr* 35:18.

Gill SK, Broussard C, Devine O, Green RF, Rasmussen SA, Reefhuis J. 2012. Association between maternal age and birth defects of unknown etiology: United States, 1997-2007. *Birt Defects Res. A. Clin. Mol. Teratol.* 94:1010-1018.

Giordano F, Abballe A, De Felip E, di Domenico A, Ferro F, Grammatico P, Ingelido AM, Marra V, Marrocco G, Vallasciani S, Figa-Talamanca I. 2010. Maternal exposures to endocrine disrupting chemicals and hypospadias in offspring. *Birt Defects Res. A. Clin. Mol. Teratol.* 88:241-250.

Hansen M, Kurinczuk JJ, Bower C, Webb S. 2002. The risk of major birth defects after intracytoplasmic sperm injection and in vitro fertilization. *N. Engl. J. Med.* 346:725-730.

Hay S, Barbano H. 1972. Independent effects of maternal age and birth order on the incidence of selected congenital malformations. *Teratology* 6:271-279.

Heller A, Rafman S, Zvagulis I, Pless IB. 1985. Birth defects and psychosocial adjustment. *Am. J. Dis. Child* 139:257-263.

Holmbeck GN, Devine KA. 2010. Psychosocial and family functioning in spina bifida. *Dev. Disabil. Res. Rev.* 16:40-46.

Hussain N, Chaghtai A, Herndon CD, Herson VC, Rosenkrantz TS, McKenna PH. 2002. Hypospadias and early gestation growth restriction in infants. *Pediatrics* 109:473-478.

International Clearinghouse for Birth Defects Monitoring Systems. 1991. Congenital malformations worldwide: a report from the International Clearinghouse for Birth Defects Monitoring Systems. New York: Elsevier Science Publishers.

Jenicek M. 2003. Foundations of evidence-based medicine. Boca Raton: Parthenon Pub. Group.

Jin L, Ye R, Zheng J, Hong S, Ren A. 2010. Secular trends of hypospadias prevalence and factors associated with it in southeast China during 1993-2005. *Birt Defects Res. A. Clin. Mol. Teratol.* 88:458-465.

Kallen B. 1988. Case control study of hypospadias, based on registry information. *Teratology* 38:45-50.

Kallen B, Bertollini R, Castilla E, Czeizel A, Knudsen LB, Martinez-Frias ML, Mastroiacovo P, Mutchinick O. 1986. A joint international study on the epidemiology of hypospadias. *Acta Paediatr Scand. Suppl.* 324:1-52.

Kallen B, Finnstrom O, Lindam A, Nilsson E, Nygren KG, Otterblad PO. 2010. Congenital malformations in infants born after in vitro fertilization in Sweden. *Birt Defects Res. A. Clin. Mol. Teratol.* 88:137-143.

Kallen B, Finnstrom O, Nygren KG, Olausson PO. 2005. In vitro fertilization (IVF) in Sweden: risk for congenital malformations after different IVF methods. *Birt Defects Res. A. Clin. Mol. Teratol.* 73:162-169.

Kallen B, Winberg J. 1979. Dealing with suspicions of malformation frequency increase. Experience with the Swedish register of congenital malformations. *Acta Paediatr Scand. Suppl.* 275:66-74.

Kallen B, Winberg J. 1982. An epidemiological study of hypospadias in Sweden. *Acta Paediatr Scand. Suppl.* 293:1-21.

Kallen K. 2002. Role of maternal smoking and maternal reproductive history in the etiology of hypospadias in the offspring. *Teratology* 66:185-191.

Kurahashi N, Murakumo M, Kakizaki H, Nonomura K, Koyanagi T, Kasai S, Sata F, Kishi R. 2004. The estimated prevalence of hypospadias in Hokkaido, Japan. *J. Epidemiol.* 14:73-77.

Leck I, Lancashire RJ. 1995. Birth prevalence of malformations in members of different ethnic groups and in the offspring of matings between them, in Birmingham, England. *J. Epidemiol. Community Health* 49:171-179.

Loane M, Dolk H, Kelly A, Teljeur C, Greenlees R, Densem J. 2011. Paper 4: EUROCAT statistical monitoring: identification and investigation of ten year trends of congenital anomalies in Europe. *Birt Defects Res. A. Clin. Mol. Teratol.* 91 Suppl 1:S31-43.

Lowry RB, Thunem NY, Silver M. 1986. Congenital anomalies in American Indians of British Columbia. *Genet Epidemiol* 3:455-467.

Lund L, Engebjerg MC, Pedersen L, Ehrenstein V, Norgaard M, Sorensen HT. 2009. Prevalence of hypospadias in Danish boys: a longitudinal study, 1977-2005. *Eur. Urol.* 55:1022-1026.

Marengo L, Farag NH, Canfield M. 2013. Body mass index and birth defects: Texas, 2005-2008. *Matern Child Health J.* 17:1898-1907.

Martinez-Frias ML, Prieto D, Prieto L, Bermejo E, Rodriguez-Pinilla E, Cuevas L. 2004. Secular decreasing trend of the frequency of hypospadias among newborn male infants in Spain. *Birt Defects Res. A. Clin. Mol. Teratol.* 70:75-81.

Mastroiacovo P, Castilla EE, Arpino C, Botting B, Cocchi G, Goujard J, Marinacci C, Merlob P, Metneki J, Mutchinick O, Ritvanen A, Rosano A. 1999. Congenital malformations in twins: an international study. *Am. J. Med. Genet.* 83:117-124.

Materna-Kiryluk A, Wisniewska K, Badura-Stronka M, Mejnartowicz J, Wieckowska B, Balcar-Boron A, Czerwionka-Szaflarska M, Gajewska E, Godula-Stuglik U, Krawczynski M, Limon J, Rusin J, Sawulicka-Oleszczuk H, Szwalkiewicz-Warowicka E, Walczak M, Latos-Bielenska A. 2009. Parental age as a risk factor for isolated congenital malformations in a Polish population. *Paediatr Perinat Epidemiol.* 23:29-40.

Matlai P, Beral V. 1985. Trends in congenital malformations of external genitalia. *Lancet* 1:108.

Mavrogenis S, Urban R, Czeizel AE. 2014. Pregnancy complications in the mothers who delivered boys with isolated hypospadias - a population-based case-control study. *J. Matern Fetal Neonatal. Med:*1-5.

McIntosh GC, Olshan AF, Baird PA. 1995. Paternal age and the risk of birth defects in offspring. *Epidemiology* 6:282-288.

Meyer KJ, Reif JS, Veeramachaneni DN, Luben TJ, Mosley BS, Nuckols JR. 2006. Agricultural pesticide use and hypospadias in eastern Arkansas. *Environ. Health Perspect* 114:1589-1595.

Mohammadzadeh A, Farhat A, Esmaieli H, Shiranzaei S. 2011. Prevalence and risk factors of hypospadias in a private hospital in northeast iran. *Iran J Pediatr* 21:497-501.

Morera AM, Valmalle AF, Asensio MJ, Chossegros L, Chauvin MA, Durand P, Mouriquand PD. 2006. A study of risk factors for hypospadias in the Rhone-Alpes region (France). *J. Pediatr. Urol.* 2:169-177.

Nassar N, Abeywardana P, Barker A, Bower C. 2010. Parental occupational exposure to potential endocrine disrupting chemicals and risk of hypospadias in infants. *Occup. Environ. Med.* 67:585-589.

Nazer J, Cifuentes L, Hubner ME, Ramirez R, Ruiz G, Pizarro MT, Nazer C, Morales I. 1992. [Epidemiologic study of factors associated with hypospadias]. *Rev. Med. Chil.* 120:244-249.

Nelson CP, Park JM, Wan J, Bloom DA, Dunn RL, Wei JT. 2005. The increasing incidence of congenital penile anomalies in the United States. *J. Urol.* 174:1573-1576.

Nissen KB, Udesen A, Garne E. 2014. Hypospadias - prevalence, birth weight and associated major congenital anomalies. *Congenit Anom* (Kyoto).

Nordenvall AS, Frisen L, Nordenstrom A, Lichtenstein P, Nordenskjold A. 2014. Population based nationwide study of hypospadias in Sweden, 1973 to 2009: incidence and risk factors. *J. Urol.* 191:783-789.

North K, Golding J. 2000. A maternal vegetarian diet in pregnancy is associated with hypospadias. The ALSPAC Study Team. Avon Longitudinal Study of Pregnancy and Childhood. *BJU Int.* 85:107-113.

Oldereid NB, Abyholm T, Tanbo T, Engelund IE, Irgens LM. 2003. [Congenital malformations in children born after assisted fertilization in Norway]. *Tidsskr Nor Laegeforen* 123:2696-2699.

Paulozzi LJ. 1999. International trends in rates of hypospadias and cryptorchidism. *Environ. Health Perspect* 107:297-302.

Paulozzi LJ, Erickson JD, Jackson RJ. 1997. Hypospadias trends in two US surveillance systems. *Pediatrics* 100:831-834.

Pierik FH, Burdorf A, Deddens JA, Juttmann RE, Weber RF. 2004. Maternal and paternal risk factors for cryptorchidism and hypospadias: a case-control study in newborn boys. *Environ. Health Perspect* 112:1570-1576.

Pinborg A, Loft A, Nyboe Andersen A. 2004. Neonatal outcome in a Danish national cohort of 8602 children born after in vitro fertilization or intracytoplasmic sperm injection: the role of twin pregnancy. *Acta Obstet. Gynecol. Scand* 83:1071-1078.

Pohl HG, Joyce GF, Wise M, Cilento BG, Jr. 2007. Cryptorchidism and hypospadias. *J. Urol.* 177:1646-1651.

Polednak AP, Janerich DT. 1983. Maternal characteristics and hypospadias: a case-control study. *Teratology* 28:67-73.

Porter MP, Faizan MK, Grady RW, Mueller BA. 2005. Hypospadias in Washington State: maternal risk factors and prevalence trends. *Pediatrics* 115:e495-499.

Ramos-Arroyo MA. 1991. Birth defects in twins: study in a Spanish population. *Acta Genet. Med. Gemellol. (Roma)* 40:337-344.

Ramos-Arroyo MA, Rodriguez-Pinilla E, Cordero JF. 1992. Maternal diabetes: the risk for specific birth defects. *Eur. J. Epidemiol.* 8:503-508.

Rankin J, Tennant PW, Stothard KJ, Bythell M, Summerbell CD, Bell R. 2010. Maternal body mass index and congenital anomaly risk: a cohort study. *Int. J. Obes* 34:1371-1380.

Reefhuis J, Honein MA. 2004. Maternal age and non-chromosomal birth defects, Atlanta--1968-2000: teenager or thirty-something, who is at risk? *Birt Defects Res. A. Clin. Mol. Teratol.* 70:572-579.

Roberts CJ, Lloyd S. 1973. Observations on the epidemiology of simple hypospadias. *Br. Med. J.* 1:768-770.

Schnack TH, Zdravkovic S, Myrup C, Westergaard T, Christensen K, Wohlfahrt J, Melbye M. 2008. Familial aggregation of hypospadias: a cohort study. *Am. J. Epidemiol* 167:251-256.

Shaw GM, Carmichael SL, Nelson V. 2002. Congenital malformations in offspring of Vietnamese women in California, 1985-97. *Teratology* 65:121-124.

Silver RI, Rodriguez R, Chang TS, Gearhart JP. 1999. In vitro fertilization is associated with an increased risk of hypospadias. *J. Urol.* 161:1954-1957.

Skriver MV, Pedersen L, Stang P, Lund L, Rothman KJ, Sorensen HT. 2004. The month of birth does not affect the risk of hypospadias. *Eur. J. Epidemiol* 19:1135-1136.

Song JW, Chung KC. 2010. Observational studies: cohort and case-control studies. *Plast Reconstr Surg.* 126:2234-2242.

Sorensen HT, Pedersen L, Norgaard M, Wogelius P, Rothman KJ. 2005. Maternal asthma, preeclampsia and risk of hypospadias. *Epidemiology* 16:806-807.

Stoll C, Alembik Y, Roth MP, Dott B. 1990. Genetic and environmental factors in hypospadias. *J. Med. Genet.* 27:559-563.

Storgaard L, Bonde JP, Olsen J. 2006. Male reproductive disorders in humans and prenatal indicators of estrogen exposure. A review of published epidemiological studies. *Reprod. Toxicol.* 21:4-15.

Sun G, Tang D, Liang J, Wu M. 2009. Increasing prevalence of hypospadias associated with various perinatal risk factors in chinese newborns. *Urology* 73:1241-1245.

Svensson J. 1979. Male hypospadias, 625 cases, associated malformations and possible etiological factors. *Acta Paediatr Scand.* 68:587-592.

Trabert B, Chodick G, Shalev V, Sella T, Longnecker MP, McGlynn KA. 2014. Gestational diabetes and the risk of cryptorchidism and hypospadias. *Epidemiology* 25:152-153.

van der Zanden LF, van Rooij IA, Feitz WF, Franke B, Knoers NV, Roeleveld N. 2012. Aetiology of hypospadias: a systematic review of genes and environment. *Hum. Reprod. Update* 18:260-283.

van Rooij IA, van der Zanden LF, Brouwers MM, Knoers NV, Feitz WF, Roeleveld N. 2013. Risk factors for different phenotypes of hypospadias: results from a Dutch case-control study. *BJU Int.* 112:121-128.

Waller DK, Shaw GM, Rasmussen SA, Hobbs CA, Canfield MA, Siega-Riz AM, Gallaway MS, Correa A. 2007. Prepregnancy obesity as a risk factor for structural birth defects. *Arch. Pediatr Adolesc. Med.* 161:745-750.

Wehrung DA, Hay S. 1970. A study of seasonal incidence of congenital malformations in the United States. *Br. J. Prev. Soc. Med.* 24:24-32.

Weidner IS, Moller H, Jensen TK, Skakkebaek NE. 1999. Risk factors for cryptorchidism and hypospadias. *J. Urol.* 161:1606-1609.

Wennerholm UB, Bergh C, Hamberger L, Lundin K, Nilsson L, Wikland M, Kallen B. 2000. Incidence of congenital malformations in children born after ICSI. *Hum. Reprod.* 15:944-948.

Winston JJ, Meyer RE, Emch ME. 2014. Geographic analysis of individual and environmental risk factors for hypospadias births. *Birt Defects Res. A. Clin. Mol. Teratol.*.

Woud SG, van Rooij IA, van Gelder MM, Olney RS, Carmichael SL, Roeleveld N, Reefhuis J. 2014. Differences in risk factors for second and third degree hypospadias in the national birth defects prevention study. *Birt Defects Res. A. Clin. Mol. Teratol.* 100:703-711.

Xu LF, Liang CZ, Lipianskaya J, Chen XG, Fan S, Zhang L, Zhou J, Tai S, Jiang CQ. 2014. Risk factors for hypospadias in China. *Asian J. Androl.*

Yoon PW, Olney RS, Khoury MJ, Sappenfield WM, Chavez GF, Taylor D. 1997. Contribution of birth defects and genetic diseases to pediatric hospitalizations. A population-based study. *Arch Pediatr Adolesc. Med.* 151:1096-1103.

In: Hypospadias
Editor: Daniel H. Preston
ISBN: 978-1-63482-023-3

Chapter 2

New Insights into Hypospadias, with Emphasis on Etiology and Epidemiology

Ali Tourchi[1,•]***, Maryam Ebadi***[2,*]***,***
Anne-Françoise Spinoit[3,#] ***and Piet Hoebeke***[3,¥]
[1]Robert D. Jeffs Division of Pediatric Urology,
James Buchanan Brady Urological Institute,
the Johns Hopkins University School of Medicine,
Baltimore, MD, US
[2]Tehran University of Medical Sciences, Iran
[3]Department of Urology, Ghent University Hospital,
Ghent, Belgium

Abstract

Hypospadias is recognized as one the most common congenital malformations in male newborns, resulting in an abnormal opening of urethral meatus. It is regarded as a multifactorial disorder in which

• E-mail: atourch1@jhmi.edu, Phone: 716-907-6994, Fax: 410-955-5358.
* E-mail: ebadi.mary20@gmail.com.
# E-mail: afspinoit@hotmail.com.
¥ E-mail: piet.hoebeke@uzgent.be.

interactions between genetics, maternal and environmental factors lead to hypoplastic development of the ventral side of the penis, either dependently or in an interaction with other factors. Various studies have pointed to contributing factors and their association with development of hypospadias. In addition epidemiologic studies have described its epidemiologic patterns. In this chapter, the authors aim to summarize various epidemiological findings, mutations and the recognized genetic aspects of the malformation, as well as the known predisposing environmental factors. Some gene-gene and gene-environment interactions have been recognized which will be discussed. Finally, the tendency of each etiologic factor to result in different phenotypes will be described.

Keywords: Hypospadias; epidemiology; gene

1. Introduction

Hypospadias is one of the most common urologic disorders encountered by pediatric urologists, with an increasing trend [1-3]. An incidence of 1/125-1/300 has been estimated [4]. It is recognized as a multifactorial disorder determined by genetic, endocrine and environmental factors which may interplay in the disease development. Understanding the exact etiology and epidemiology seems mandatory for both prevention and application of correct therapeutic approaches, leading to better outcome and quality of life. Despite various studies on epidemiology and etiology, a review on this aspects is not published. In this review, we seek to integrate the actual epidemiologic and genetic basis of hypospadias, up until October 2013, in order to obtain a new insight in the pathophysiology of this malformation.

2. Epidemiology

The incidence of hypospadias is on the rise in the USA [5, 2]; with various between-state differences in prevalence [5]. Briefly the prevalence rate is reported to be higher in Arkansas compared to reports from other states. Between 2002-2006, 83.0 per 10,000 live-birth cases were reported from Arkansas, compared to 62.2 for Utah, 61.6 for North Carolina, 56.8 for Georgia, 54.0 for Texas, 40.5 for Oklahoma and 37.9 for Iowa [6]. According to epidemiologic studies, the incidence and severity of hypospadias in small for gestational age (SGA) newborns is increased [7-8]. A retrospective cohort study revealed an increased ratio of mild to severe hypospadias in newborns with SGA compared to the population with normal birth weight; the prevalence of SGA in patients with hypospadias is significantly greater than the 11% incidence observed in newborns with normal weight [8]. Huisima et al. [8] stated a 65% prevalence of severe hypospadias in SGA newborns; similarly, Yinon et al. [9] observed a 62% ratio in pregnancies with intrauterine growth restriction (IUGR). In addition, white ethnicity is described as a potential risk factor for the development of hypospadias [10]. Similarly, Canon et al. [5] reported greater incidence of first degree hypospadias in white non-Hispanic maternal ethnicity. Conversely, lower prevalence was detected in African-Americans and Hispanics in the same study. It is postulated that the increased prevalence of first, second and third degree hypospadias in recent years may be due to improved knowledge and recognition of this congenital malformation [5]; nonetheless, Nordenvall et al. described that the increased incidence is independent of better detection [2]. Table I summarizes the incidence rate according to various studies.

3. Etiology

No solid etiology for hypospadias has been delineated in the literature. It is described as a multifactorial disorder, consisting of genetic, endocrine and environmental factors, which may independently or in combination, disrupt normal formation of external genitalia; a cocktail of etiologies may interact in its pathogenesis. In addition, the exact etiology in isolated cases cannot be elucidated [11]. Interaction between several genes and environmental factors have been determined [12]. Nonetheless, recent studies have shed light on the etiology of this congenital malformation.

3.1. Maternal Factors

Maternal-placental factors are independently correlated with the development of hypospadias [8]; it is suggested that some cases of severe hypospadias may be causally related to maternal-placental factors [13, 7]. Yinon et al. [9] described a correlation between severities of IUGR and hypospadias.

In a study by Huisma et al. [8] risk factors for SGA including prematurity, preeclampsia and placental insufficiency were independently associated with the incidence of hypospadias.

Table I. The incidence of hypospadias based on various studies

Study	Year	Incidence	Location	Ref.
Paulozzi et al.	1970	20.2 per 10,000	USA	[1]
Elliott et al.	1985	47 per 10,000	USA (state of California)	[2]
Paulozzi et al.	1993	39.7 per 10,000	USA	[1]
Nordenvall et al.	1973-2009	1973-1990: 4.5 per 1,000 1990-2009: 8 per 1,000	Sweden	[3]
Gallentine et al.	1990-1998	0.7%	USA	[4]
Pierik et al.	2002	38 per 10,000	Netherlands and Finland	[5]
Elliott et al.	2006	57 per 10,000	USA (state of California)	[2]
Akin et al.	2007-2008	93.7 per 10,000	Turkey (Istanbul)	[6]
Ghirri et al.	2009	3.066 per 1,000	Italy	[7]
Huang et al.	1997-2008	33.8 per 10,000	Taiwan	[8]

[1]Paulozzi L. J., Erickson J. D., Jackson R. J. (1997) Hypospadias trends in two US surveillance systems. Pediatrics, 100(5):831-4.

[2]Elliott C. S., Halpern M. S., Paik J., et al (2011) Epidemiologic trends in penile anomalies and hypospadias in the state of California, 1985–2006. J. Ped. Urol., 7(3):294-8.

[3]Nordenvall A. S., Frisén L., Nordenström A., et al (2014) A Population-Based Nationwide Study of Hypospadias in Sweden, 1973–2009: Incidence and Risk Factors. J. Urol., 191(3):783-9.

[4]Gallentine M. L., Morey A. F., Thompson Jr. I. M. (2001) Hypospadias: a contemporary epidemiologic assessment. Urology, 57(4):788-90.

[5]Pierik F. H., Burdorf A., Nijman J. R., de Muinck Keizer-Schrama S. M., Juttmann R., Weber R.F. (2002) A high hypospadias rate in The Netherlands. Human reproduction, 17(4):1112-5.

[6]Akin Y., Ercan O., Telatar B., Tarhan F., Comert S. (2011) Hypospadias in Istanbul: Incidence and risk factors. Pediatrics Int., 53(5):754-60.

[7]Ghirri P., Scaramuzzo R. T., Bertelloni S., et al. (2009) Prevalence of hypospadias in Italy according to severity, gestational age and birthweight: an epidemiological study. Ital. J. Pediatr., 35:18.

[8]Huang W.-Y., Chen Y.-F., Guo Y.-J., Lan C.-F., Chang H.-C., Chen S.-C. et al. Epidemiology of hypospadias and treatment trends in Taiwan: a nationwide study. The Journal of urology, 2011;185(4):1449-54.

In addition, maternal hypertension, prematurity and oligohydraminos were more prevalent among patients with severe hypospadias compared to mild cases [8]. It is hypothesized that placental insufficiency contributes to the development of hypospadias through its interactions with other risk factors, namely LBW and maternal hypertension as a causal factor, and with multiple pregnancies as a resultant [14]. Maternal obesity, primiparity, multiparity and twin pregnancies lead to disturbance in androgen/estrogen balance, especially in first and twin pregnancies; hence disturbing normal male genital formation [15]. The risk of developing this malformation is doubled in twins and first-born children [14]. It is believed that since first born children are more prone to SGA, their greater risk could be explained [16]. With respect to twins, the sex of the twins is known to influence the risk of hypospadias; a 1.9 times greater risk is observed in male-male twins in comparison with the male pair in male-female twins. Overall, placenta interactions in multiple births is recognized as the underlying cause twins [16].

Debate exists on the relationship between maternal age and abnormal male genitalia development; Carmichael et al. [17] and Carlson et al. [18] described a positive correlation between maternal age with the incidence and severity of hypospadias. Similarly, a positive linear correlation has been described between maternal age and the risk of hypospadias [10]. Nevertheless, no significant association was found in another study [12]. Interestingly, low maternal education has been associated with increased risk of hypospadias [19]; however, the mechanism through which it exerts its influence was not fully described. We hypothesize that education level could act indirectly by exerting its deleterious effect on other maternal factors including preeclampsia and prematurity.

Preexisting maternal diabetes is also recognized as a potential maternal risk factor; moreover, mild gestational diabetes was also significantly correlated to the malformation [20]. Other maternal diseases including epilepsy (possibly through the medications administered), renal failure, asthma and influenza during the first semester may lead to an increased risk [16]. Moreover, Klip et al. [21] observed that women exposed to DES during their fetal period are at a greater risk of giving birth to boys with hypospadias.

Various studies have investigated the impact of assisted human reproduction on the development of genitalia abnormalities. In vitro fertilization(IVF) and IVF/ intracytoplasmic injection (ICSI) are indirectly associated with increased hypospadias rate [10], possibly via augmentation of LBW and preterm labor [22]. A 5-fold increased risk of hypospadias with an incidence of 1.46% has been observed in male offsprings conceived by IVF [23].

Olson et al. [24] stated that the exact mechanism through which IVF leads to hypospadias remains unknown, whereas silver et al. proposed that progesterone administration during the IVF procedure may account for the increased risk. In addition, higher maternal age in the IVF group, may indirectly lead to increased hypospadias incidence [23].

3.2. Environmental Factors

Environmental risk factors have been hypothesized to act in concert with genetic factors, contributing to the development of hypospadias. Various environmental risk factors have been recognized in this regard including the trans-generational effects of diethylstilbestrol, fertility treatments and environmental endocrine disruptions (EEDs) [25]. Environmental endocrine disruptors such as 2,3,7,8-tetrachlorodibenzop-dioxin, are increasingly and uncontrolled released into the environment, adding to the prevalence of hypospadias [26]. EDC exposure during early fetal life is recognized to increase the risk of hypospadias development by alteration, mimicking or blocking the action of endocrine hormones [27]. Rocheleau et al. described parental endocrine disruption due to exposure to pesticides, which eventually manifested as hypospadias in the offspring [27]; however, no association was found in another study [28]. On the other hand, phthalate-induced alterations in male reproductive development have been well elucidated. Hypospadias, as a phenotype of 'testicular dysgenesis syndrome' is predicated on reduction in testosterone production by the fetal Leydig cell. Li et al. [29] studied the dose-related effect of maternal exposure to di-(2-ethylhexyl) phthalate (DEHP) plasticizer on external genitalia in adult male offspring rats, and described a positive correlation between the dose of DEHP and the severity of hypospadias in male rats. However, the observed association merits further investigation in human patients. Klinfelter et al. examined the pathways through which DEHP exposure leads to gonadal dysgenesis, and reported that all proteins involved are part of a network in which each protein is regulated directly or indirectly by estradiol [30]. Maternal exposure to diethylstilbestrol is also linked to abnormal male genitalia development [31]. Based on the hypothesis that endocrine disruptors play an etiologic role in the development of hypospadias, Choi et al. studied various endocrine disruptors including 5 phthalates ((DEHP), di-n-butyl-phthalate (DBP), mono-(2- ethylhexyl) phthalate (MEHP), mono-n-butyl-phthalate (MBP) and phthalic acid (PA)), 2 alkylphenols (n-nonylphenol (n-NP) and t-octylphenol (t-OP)) and bisphenol A. As assessed by concentrations of the above mentioned chemical in urine and plasma specimen of both patients and control group, DEHP (P = 0.006) and n-NP (P = 7.26e-6) in the urine samples, as well as PA (P = 0.009) and BPA (P = 7.22e-10) in plasma samples showed a significant association with hypospadias. To investigate possible metastasis of endocrine disruptors from the mother to child, concentrations in the urine and plasma of the offspring were compared to those of the mother. Nonetheless, a correlation was not found in this regard [32].

Gestational exposure to estrogenic compounds increases the risk of hypospadias. On the other hand, high consumption of total phytoestrogenes, daidzein, genistein, glycetin, secoisolariciresinol, total isoflavones and lignans, which have potential impacts on estrogen matabolism, leads to risk reduction [33]. Studies have also pointed to family history as a potential risk factor in the development of this congenital abnormality [34]; 14% and 8% recurrence risk is observed with an involved sibling or father, respectively [35]. Moreover, environmental pollutants with estrogenic or antiandrogenic properties are also known to contribute in the etiology [25]. It is well established that increased exposure to estrogen in utero may impair Leydig cell development, suppress testosterone production or androgen receptor expression, leading to male reproductive abnormalities including hypospadias [36].

3.3. Dietary and Pharmaceutical Factors

Various dietary nutrients and medications during pregnancy are recognized to play a pivotal role in the development of this malformation.

Maternal diet during pregnancy has been correlated with hypospadias development in various studies. Christensen et al. evaluated the effect of maternal organic diet during pregnancy on the development of hypospadias in the offspring. Low consumption of organic food and consuming their non-organic alternatives were associated with greater risk. In addition, low rate of butter and cheese consumption led to increased odds ratio; all of which bring up the notion that life style behaviors relevant to choosing organics can be associated with hypospadias. It is described in the literature that conventional diets contain pesticides which have resided in the feedstuff supplied to nonorganic dairy cattle transformed through milk; the greater the fat content of these dairy products, the higher the probability that pesticides would concentrate in these products with endocrine disrupting properties; hence increasing the risk of hypospadias [37]. With respect to animal products, no association with hypospadias has been found. In addition, diet quality or intake of iron supplements and other nutrients influencing estrogen metabolism has no established effect [38]. However, North et al. [39] described that since vegetarians are at a greater risk of exposure to phytoestrogens, the risk of hypospadias is increased in their offspring. Between 1999-2003, increased cocoa consumption in early pregnancy was significantly correlated to the incidence of hypospadias [40].

Smoking and alcohol have a divergent effect on the incidence of posterior hypospadias. Rooij et al. [12] described an increased risk in some cases, whereas reduction in some other cases were reported. Remarkably, most studies on the impact of smoking and alcohol consumption haven't found a significant correlation [41-42, 19].

Consumption of hormone containing contraceptives after conception is significantly associated with elevated risk [12]. In addition, administration of antiepileptic medication during pregnancy enhances the probability; a dose dependent pattern has been described between the consumption of valporate during the first semester and the risk of hypospadias development. Therefore, it is believed that reduction in valporate dose in early pregnancy may significantly reduce the risk [43].

Interestingly, debate persists on the impact of β-blockers during early pregnancy; nonetheless, a recent meta-analysis reported that β-blocker consumption during the first semester has no significant effect on the development of hypospadias in the offspring [44]. A brief of the mentioned etiologic factors has been summarized in Table II.

3.4. Genetics

During recent years, genetic abnormalities have been described as one of the main etiologic factors. Huisma et al. performed the first genome wide association study on hypospadias. They surmised that increased incidence of hypospadias in SGA infants might be due to genetic syndromes or multiple congenital abnormalities [8].

To name a few, 9P partial monosomy leads to the development of various genitourinary abnormalities including hypospadias in the male fetus. Quinonez et al. described that the 9p24.3 location, specifically DMRT1, is responsible for gonadal dysgenesis observed in these patients [45].

In addition, a multitude of genes are recognized to play a fundamental role in the development of hypospadias including WT1, SF1, BMP4, BMP7, HOXA4, HOXB6, AR, FGF8, FGFR2, HSD3B2,SRD5A2, ATF3, MAMLD1, MID1, BNC2, ESR1, ESR2,ATF3, DGKK, CYP1A1, GSTM1, GSTT1, CTGF, CYR61 and EGF [31]. Patients with hypospadias manifest greater androgen receptor (AR) gene methylation in their foreskin [46]. AR is a steroid receptor and its gene is located on Xq11-12 position of the X chromosome. Various polymorphisms in the AR gene have been studied including CAG and GGN polymorphisms [47]. Parado-Busamante et al. [47] assessed CAG/GGN polymorphism in patients with non-severe and severe isolated cases, in whom hormonal status was normal; AR of patients with hypospadias revealed longer CAG alleles. It is deemed that abnormal variations in the AR gene sequence impair the receptor's transcriptional activity, resulting in the development of hypospadias [48]. In the same line, Palazzolo et al. [49] reported that abnormal length of the two polymorphic zones in the AR gene formed by consecutive repeats of CAG and GGN triplets alter the transcriptional activity of the AR gene [49]. An inverse correlation has been found between the number of CAG repeats and the transcriptional activity of AR [50]. Nonetheless, the molecular mechanism beyond this association remains to be elucidated. Parada-Bustamante et al. [47] demonstrated that the interaction between AR protein and co-activating or co-repressing molecules is directly affected by the length of the polyglutamine tract [47]. A multitude of studies have demonstrated that a long length of CAG or GCN polymorphisms in the AR gene may play an etiologic role in the development of isolated hypospadias [47, 51-52]. Precisely, lengths>40 repeats lead to the aggregation of AR proteins in cells through misfolding of the AR protein [53]. Two CpG sites in AR, 1 in BMP4 and 2 in CTGF genes are reported to be significantly associated with hypospadias, surmising an etiologic role for these genes via epigenetic mechanisms [54]. A novel AR mutation, c.2214T>G;p.Ile738Met, has been identified in patients with testicular dysgenesis syndrome including hypospadias. Approximately, 50% reduction in AR-induced transcriptional activity was found on functional analysis, resulting in elevated LH and T as a consequence of decreased AR signaling [55].

Mutations in genes involved in the androgen synthesis, 5α-reductase type II gene [48] and 3β-hydroxysteriod dehydrogenase type II gene [56] have been observed in patients with isolated hypospadias. Moreover, partial organ insensitivity and 5α-reductase type II deficiency are described in some cases [57].

Table II. Maternal and pharmaceutical factors involved in the pathogenesis of hypospadias

Study	Factor	Reference
Huisma et al. 2001 Ghirri et al .2009, Yamazaki et al. 2006 Yinin et al. 2010	SGA *	[1-4]
Akre et al., 2008 Hussain et al. 2002	SGA risk factors including : prematurity, preeclampsia, multiple gestations placental insufficiency , Oligohydraminos	[5-6]
Porter et al., 2005	Maternal age	[7]
Mouriquand et al., 2007	White ethnicity	[8]
Pierik et al., 2004	Maternal education	[9]
Hjartaker et al. 2007	Maternal obesity, Primiparity, multiparity ,twin pregnancies	[10]
Main et al. 2010	Maternal diabetes	[11]
Klip et al.2002	Maternal exposure to DES* during their own fetal period	[12]
Schnack et al. 2010	Family history	[13]
Baskin et al. 2001 Gaspari et al. 2011 Li et al. 2012	Pollutants containing estrogenic or antiandrogenic properties	[14-16]
Porter et al., 2005 Bang et al., 2013	IVF/ ICSI*	[7] [17]
Norgil Damgaard et al., 2002	Low maternal consumption of organic food	[18]
Giannandrea et al.,2009	increased cocoa consumption	[19]
North et al., 2000	Vegetarianism and consumption of phytoestrogens	[20]
Rooij et al.,2013	Consumption of hormone containing contraceptives after conception	[21]
Vajda et al., 2013	Antiepileptic medication during pregnancy	[22]

SGA: small for gestational age; DES: diethylstilbestrol; IVF: In vitro fertilization; ICSI: intra-cytoplasmic injection.

[1]Huisma F., Thomas M., Armstrong L. (2013) Severe hypospadias and its association with maternal-placental factors. American Journal of Medical Genetics Part A, 161(9):2183-7.

[2]Gatti J., Kirsch A., Troyer W., et al. (2001) Increased incidence of hypospadias in small-for-gestational age infants in a neonatal intensive-care unit. BJU international, 87(6):548-50.

[3]Yamazaki H., Yamazaki A., Nagayama Y. (2006) The association between hypospadias in neonates and intrauterine growth retardation. J. Japan Soci. Perinat. Neonat. Med., 42(1):25-9.

[4]Yinon Y., Proctor L. K., Kelly E. N., et al. (2010) Hypospadias in males with intrauterine growth restriction due to placental insufficiency: the placental role in the embryogenesis of male external genitalia. American Journal of Medical Genetics, Part A, 152(1):75-83.

[5]Hussain N., Chaghtai A., Herndon C. A., et al. (2002) Hypospadias and early gestation growth restriction in infants. Pediatrics, 109(3):473-8.

[6]Huisma F., Thomas M., Armstrong L. (2013). Severe hypospadias and its association with maternal-placental factors. Am. J. Med. Genet., Part A, 161(9): 2183-7.

[7].Porter M. P., Faizan M. K., Grady R. W., et al. (2005) Hypospadias in Washington State: maternal risk factors and prevalence trends. Pediatrics, 115(4):e495-e9.

[8]Pierre Mouriquand (2007) Dialogues in Pediatric Urology, J. Ped. Urol., 28.

[9]Pierik F. H., Burdorf A., Deddens J. A., et al (2004) Maternal and paternal risk factors for cryptorchidism and hypospadias: a case–control study in newborn boys. Environ. Health Perspect., 112(15):1570.

[10]Hjartaker A., Ballard-Barbash R., Veierød M. B., et al. (2008) 17-beta-Estradiol in relation to age at menarche and adult obesity in premenopausal women. Hum. Reprod., 23(4):919-27.

[11]Main K. M., Skakkebæk N. E., Virtanen H. E., et al (2010) Genital anomalies in boys and the environment. Best Prac. Res. Clin. Endocrinol. Metabolism, 24(2):279-89.

[12]Klip H., Verloop J., van Gool J. D., et al. (2002) Hypospadias in sons of women exposed to diethylstilbestrol in utero: a cohort study. Lancet, 359(9312):1102-7.

[13]Schnack T. H., Poulsen G., Myrup C., et al. (2010) Familial coaggregation of cryptorchidism, hypospadias, and testicular germ cell cancer: a nationwide cohort study. J. Natl. Cancer Inst., 102(3):187-92.

[14]Baskin L. S., Himes K., Colborn T. (2001) Hypospadias and endocrine disruption: is there a connection? Environ. Health Perspect., 109(11):1175.

[15]Gaspari L., Paris F., Jandel C., et al. (2011) Prenatal environmental risk factors for genital malformations in a population of 1442 French male newborns: a nested case–control study. Human Reproduct., 26(11):3155-62.

[16]Li M., Qiu L., Zhang Y., et al. (2013) Dose-related effect by maternal exposure to di-(2-ethylhexyl) phthalate plasticizer on inducing hypospadiac male rats. Environ. Toxicol. Pharmacol., 35(1):55-60.

[17]Bang J. K., Lyu S. W., Choi J., et al. (2013) Does infertility treatment increase male reproductive tract disorder? Urology, 81(3):644-8.

[18]Norgil Damgaard I., Maria Main K., Toppari J., et al (2002) Impact of exposure to endocrine disrupters< i> inutero</i> and in childhood on adult reproduction. Best Prac. Res. Clin. Endocrinol. Metabolism, 16(2):289-309.

[19]Giannandrea F. (2009). Correlation analysis of cocoa consumption data with worldwide incidence rates of testicular cancer and hypospadias. Int. J. Environ. Res. Public Health, 6(2):568-78.

[20]North K., Golding J. (2000) A maternal vegetarian diet in pregnancy is associated with hypospadias. BJU Int., 85(1):107-13.

[21]Rooij I. A., Zanden L. F., Brouwers M. M., et al (2013) Risk factors for different phenotypes of hypospadias: results from a Dutch case–control study. BJU Int., 112(1):121-8.

[22]Vajda F. J., O'Brien T. J., Graham J. E., et al. (2013) Dose dependence of fetal malformations associated with valproate. Neurology, 81(11):999-1003.

Diacylglycerol kinase kappa (DGKK) gene, located on chromosome X, plays an established role [58-59]. DGKK mRNA is exclusively expressed in the testis and the placenta [60]. As established in the literature, murine males with hypospadias also express DGKK in their reproductive tract tissue during embryogenesis [61]. In addition, the gene is expressed in the preputial skin of healthy newborn males [59]. An increased risk for mild to moderate phenotypes are observed in the presence of single-nucleotide polymorphysims (SNPs) of the DGKK gene [58]. SNPs, rs1934179 (SNP22, intronic) and rs7063116 (SNP27, in the 5= upstream region) are correlated to the development of modest and moderate hypospadias [59]. Moreover, haplotypes have stronger association compared to individual SNPs [58]. The association of multiple SNPs together plays a more predominant effect on the risk of hypospadias compared to a single SNP [58]. SNP7 is modestly associated with mild to moderate variants; a 2-3 fold increased risk is observed in the adjusted analysis [58]. SNP in SRD5A2 leads to decreased formation of dihyrotestosterone (DHT) [62]. Noteworthy, the exact underlying mechanism through which DGKK gene plays an etiologic role remains to be unveiled.

SNPs in endocrine related genes including those encoding ESR, ESR2, ATF3 and SRD5A2 are involved in hypospadias development [63-64]. ATF3, an estrogen responsive gene, and SRD5A2, a gene encoding an enzyme which converts circulating testosterone in the genital tubercle to the more potent DHT, are upregulated in these patients [65, 62].

By applying epigenic approaches using DNA methylation, Choudhry et al. [54] revealed that genes such as SCARB1 and MYBPH contribute to the development of hypospadias [54]. SCARB1, in collaboration with some other genes, has been found to play a critical role in di(n-butyl) phthalate induced suppression of steroidogenesis [66]. It is reported that methylation of CpG site cg23556238 in SCARB1 is increased by two-folds in children with hypospadias, as compared with normal children, conferring to the downregulation of SCARB1 gene in hypospadias [67].

Li et al. [68] evaluated the expression of c-Jun N-terminal kinase (JNK) 1/2 in human hypospadiac tissue compared with that in normal penile tissue, and reported JNK upregulation in hypospadias patients, which may be associated with mesenchymal cell migration in the process of external male genitalia defect development.

MAMLD1 (mastermind-like domain containing 1) is recently recognized as a causative gene for 46,XY disorders of sex development, including hypospadias. Nonetheless, a handful of 6 patients with hypospadias have been reported with microdeletions in the MAMLD1 gene, and another 6 cases have been reported with definitive mutations. In addition, increased specific MAMLD1 cSNP(s) and haplotype may constitute a susceptibility factor for hypospadias. In mouse model, it was found to be expressed in fetal Sertoli and Leydig cells around the critical period of sex development. In addition, transient Mamld1 knockdown resulted in significantly reduced testosterone production due to compromised 17α-hydroxylation and Cyp17a1 expression in murine Leydig tumor cells. MAMLD1 is regulated by steroidogenic factor 1 (SF-1). It is suggested that MAMLD1 mutation leads to hypospadias through compromised testosterone production around the critical period of sex development [69]. In mice model, deletion of the gene encoding SF-1 (Nr5a1) of steroidogenic factor-1 (SF-1) (Ad4BP, NR5A1),a nuclear receptor that plays a key role in adrenal and reproductive development and function, results in severe developmental defects of the adrenal gland and gonad, including hypospadias [70]. In a recent study by Carmichael et al. several genes involved in sex hormone biosynthesis and metabolism, namely *CYP3A4*, *HSD17B3*, *HSD3B1*, *STARD3*, *SRD5A2* and in *STS* were associated with hypospadias risk [71].

The human luteinizing hormone/chorionic gonadotropin receptor (LHCGR) plays a fundamental role in male and female reproductive physiology. Mild forms of LH resistance resulting from inactivating mutations of the LHCGR lead to the development of hypospadias [72]. Table III summarizes the genes involved in the development of this congenital malformation.

3.5. Hormonal Abnormalities

Normal genital differentiation is mostly dependent on fetal androgens [54]. Impaired androgenic secretion or action during the development of external genitalia in fetal period plays an etiologic role in the development of this congenital abnormality [73, 47]. During fetal period, androgens are produced by fetal testes, and play a crucial role in the development of male genitalia during weeks 8-14 [74]. Dihydrotestosterone, the androgen which plays the most important role in the development of external genitalia, acts through AR [73].

Impaired androgen production leads to the development of isolated hypospadias [47, 75].

3.6. Interactions between Genetics, Environment And Parental Factors

As elucidated in the literature, impaired underlying mechanisms of fetal androgens during development result in disturbed epigenic programming of gene expression [54].

Table III. Genetic modifications associated with the development of hypospadias

Study	Genetic involvement	Ref.
Parada-Bustamante et al. ,2012	Androgen receptor CAG and GGN polymorphisms	[1]
Lottrup et al.,2013	c.2214T>G;p.Ile738Met mutation in the androgen receptor	[2]
Wang et al., 2004	Mutation in 5α-reductase type II gene	[3]
Codner et al., 2004	Mutations in 3β-hydroxysteriod dehydrogenase type II gene	[4]
Choudhry et al., 2012	Two CpG sites in AR 1 CpG in BMP4 2 CpGs in CTGF genes	[5]
Quinonez et al., 2013	9P partial monosomy (9p24.3 location, specifically DMRT1)	[6]
Carmichael et al., 2012 Van der Zanden et al., 2010	SNPs* rs1934179 and rs7063116 in the diacylglycerol kinase kappa (DGKK) gene located on X chromosome	[7-8]
Beleza-Meireles et al., 2008 Wang et al., 2008	SNPs in ESR, ESR2, ATF3 and SRD5A2 genes	[9-10]
Choudhry et al., 2012	Mutations in SCARB1 and MYBPH genes	[5]
Van der Zanden et al. , 2012	WT1, SF1, BMP4, BMP7, HOXA4, HOXB6, AR, FGF8, FGFR2, HSD3B2,SRD5A2, ATF3, MAMLD1, MID1, BNC2, ESR1, ESR2,ATF3, DGKK, CYP1A1, GSTM1, GSTT1, CTGF, CYR61 and EGF	[11]
Ogata et al., 2013	Microdeletions in the MAMLD1 gene	[12]
Latronico et al.,2012	Mutations of the LHCGR	[13]
El-Khairi et al., 2012	Deletion in Nr5a1 gene (encoding SF-1)	[14]
Carmichael et al., 2013	*Mutations in CYP3A4, HSD17B3, HSD3B1, STARD3, SRD5A2* and in *STS*	[15]
Li et al.,2013	JNK upregulation	[16]

*SNP: single-nucleotide polymorphysims.

[1]Parada-Bustamante A., Lardone M. C., Madariaga M., et al. (2012) Androgen receptor CAG and GGN polymorphisms in boys with isolated hypospadias. J. Ped. Endocrinol. Metabolism, 25(1-2):157-62.

[2]Lottrup G., Jørgensen A., Nielsen J. E., et al. (2013) Identification of a novel androgen receptor mutation in a family with multiple components compatible with the testicular dysgenesis syndrome. J. Clin. Endocrinol. Metabolism, 98(6):2223-9.

[3]Wang Y., Li Q., Xu J., et al. (2004) Mutation analysis of five candidate genes in Chinese patients with hypospadias. Eur. J. Hum. Genet., 12(9):706-12.

[4]Codner E. O. C., Iniguez G., Boric M. A., et al. (2004) Molecular study of the 3 beta-hydroxysteroid dehydrogenase gene type II in patients with hypospadias. J. Clin. Endocrinol. Metab., 89.

[5]Choudhry S., Deshpande A., Qiao L., et al. (2012) Genome-wide DNA Methylation Profiling of CpG Islands in Hypospadias. J. Urol., 188(4suppl.):1450-5.

[6]Quinonez S. C., Park J. M., Rabah R., et al. (2013) 9p partial monosomy and disorders of sex development: Review and postulation of a pathogenetic mechanism. American Journal of Medical Genetics, Part A, 161(8):1882-96.

[7]Carmichael S. L., Mohammed N., Ma C., et al. (2013) Diacylglycerol Kinase K Variants Impact Hypospadias in a California Study Population. J. Urol., 189(1):305-11.
[8]van der Zanden L. F., van Rooij I. A., Feitz W. F., et al. (2010) Common variants in DGKK are strongly associated with risk of hypospadias. Nat. Genet., 43(1):48-50.
[9]Beleza-Meireles A., Töhönen V., Söderhäll C., et al. (2008) Activating transcription factor 3: a hormone responsive gene in the etiology of hypospadias. Eur. J. Endocrinol., 158(5):729-39.
[10]Wang M. H., Baskin L. S. (2008) Endocrine disruptors, genital development, and hypospadias. J. Androl., 29(5):499-505.
[11]Van der Zanden L., van Rooij I., Feitz W., et al. (2012) Aetiology of hypospadias: a systematic review of genes and environment. Hum. Reprod. Update, 18(3):260-83.
[12]Ogata T., Sano S., Nagata E., Kato F., Fukami M., editors. MAMLD1 and 46, XY Disorders of Sex Development. Seminars in reproductive medicine; 2012: Thieme Medical Publishers.
[13]Latronico A. C. A. I. (2012). Inactivating mutations of the human luteinizing hormone receptor in both sexes. Semin. Reprod. Med., 30(5):382-6.
[14]El-Khairi R., Achermann J. C., editors. Steroidogenic Factor-1 and Human Disease. Seminars in reproductive medicine; 2012: Thieme Medical Publishers.
[15]Carmichael S., Witte J., Ma C., et al. (2014) Hypospadias and variants in genes related to sex hormone biosynthesis and metabolism. Andrology, 2(1):130-7.
[16]Li M., Qiu L., Lin T., et al. (2013) c-Jun N-Terminal Kinase is Upregulated in Patients With Hypospadias. Urology, 81(1):178-83.

Genetics, maternal and environmental factors interact with one another in the development of hypospadias, and may explicate the genetic non-replication between various studies [62].

The intrauterine environment may be affected by maternal genotype, preceded by modulation in the risk of hypospadias. On the other hand, genomic imprinting may influence the risk; as it may lead to greater expression of the copy derived from one parent [76]. With respect to the interaction between the presence of SNPs in SRD5A2 and exogenous estrogen exposure during pregnancy, Ven der Zanden et al. revealed that only fetus carrying the SNP in SRD5A2 genome have an increased risk of hypospadias once exposed to exogenous estrogen during pregnancy [62]; exogenous estrogen exposure in patients with SNP variant in SRD5A2 leads to substitution of valine with leucine (V89L), followed by reduction in the enzyme's capability in producing dihydrotestosterone by 30% [62]. On the other hand, the presence of SNP in SRD5A2 modulates the risk of hypospadias in cases with placental insufficiency including maternal hypertension and preeclampsia [62]. It is recognized that SNP in ATF3 increases the risk of hypospadias in cases with maternal infection or inflammation during gestation [62]. Surprisingly, only ESR1 with maternal origin is associated with increased risk of hypospadias, since it is more fully expressed [62]. Abnormalities in fetal androgens act through mechanisms which disrupt epigenic programming of gene expression during the development of fetal genitalia, resulting in hypospadias [54]. Epigenic mechanisms involving various CpG sites in AR, BMP4 and CTGF have pertinent roles in this regard [54]. Noteworthy, various factors interact in the influence of EEDs in hypospadias development including the individual's susceptibility and developmental stage, as well as the dose and type of the EED [31]. Qin et al. described an association between the incidence of hypospadias and SNPs in all 5 genes involved in EED metabolism [77]. A meaningful correlation has been described between the incidence of hypospadias and the aryl hydrocarbon receptor nuclear translocator 2 (ARNT2) gene, which is found to be implicated in the dioxin signaling pathway [78]. Dioxin binds to AHR, preceded by transactivation of several target genes and modulation of estrogen receptor signaling. Therefore, the involvement of specific alleles of genes involved in the dioxin signaling pathway results in susceptibility to EEDs and eventually leads to the development of undermasculinized genitaliahave been established [79]. Moreover, SNPs in CYP1A2, NR1I2 and CYP17A1 are also observed in patients with hypospadias; CYP1A2 and NR1I2 play a crucial role in EED metabolism, whereas CYP17A1 encodes one of the key enzymes involved in estrogen biosynthesis. Possible synergic interactions between SNPs in ARNT2 and those in the four other genes predisposing to hypospadias have been implicated. Therefore, complex gene–gene and gene-environmental interactions increase the risk of EED-induced hypospadias [77].

4. Predisposition to Different Phenotypes of Hypospadias

Depending on the location of the urethral opening along the penis or scrotum, hypospadias is subdivided into anterior, posterior, middle and distal forms [5]. Various etiologic factors are involved in the development of each phenotype as discussed below.

The impact of various etiologic factors during different embryonic stages leads to the development of diverse phenotypes [12]. However, the underlying etiologic cause leading to various hypospadias phenotypes is not fully delineated. During embryogenesis, fusion of labioscrotal swellings leads to the formation of the scrotum, and close folding of the urethra forms the penile urethra. Specific phenotypes of hypospadias are formed through disturbance in one of these embryonic processes. During different stages of gestation, genetic and environmental factors exert different impacts on the development of male external genitalia, resulting in various phenotypes [12].

Since the majority of familial hypospadias are found to be anterior or middle phenotypes [41], genetic predisposition is found to play a predominant role in the development of these variants, whereas, pregnancy-related risk factors including primiparity, preterm labor and SGA are mostly correlated with posterior phenotypes [12].

DGKK gene plays an established role in the development of anterior and middle phenotypes. Contrariwise, its role in the development of posterior hypospadias is not fully determined [59].

Overall maternal risk factors most significantly contribute to the development of posterior phenotypes. De-novo mutations and mother-derived mutations are described in posterior phenotypes [31], which might also count for the lower frequency of family history in this subgroup. Moreover, posterior hypospadias is significantly correlated to pregnancy-related factors [12]; SGA is a significant risk factor for the development of posterior hypospadias. Preeclampsia is mostly related to posterior phenotypes [41]. In addition, primiparity and multiple pregnancies are associated with increased incidence of this subgroup [31]. Moreover, among SGA patients developing hypospadias, proximal hypospadias is reported to be more significantly associated with maternal hypertension, oligohydraminos and premature delivery, in comparison with patients with distal hypospadias [8]. Interestingly, twins and first born children have a four and seven fold increased risk of posterior hypospadias, respectively [12]. With respect to maternal medications during gestational period, consumption of hormone-based contraceptives after conception mostly contributes to the formation of middle and posterior variants [8].

Clomiphene exposure during pregnancy exclusively contributes to the development of penoscrotal hypospadias, conferring to the role of estrogen activity in posterior variants [80]. Conversely, Reefhius et al. found no significant association between penoscrotal hypospadias and clomiphene exposure after adjustment for confounding factors such as maternal age and socioeconomic status [80]. Finally, maternal age >35 years and white non-Hispanic maternal ethnicity only led to greater incidence in first degree hypospadias [5, 16].

Conclusion

In general, hypospadias is a congenital malformation with a variety of etiologic and epidemiologic basis, acting dependently or independently throughout fetal period, eventually leading to this malformation in male newborns. A comprehensive knowledge and thorough understanding of its etiology and epidemiology would aid obstetrics and pediatric urologists in early diagnosis, better recognition and hopefully prevention of this worldwide increasing disorder. This study was stopped in November 2013.

Conflict of Interest

None.

Source of Funding

None.

References

[1] Paulozzi L. J. (1999) International trends in rates of hypospadias and cryptorchidism. *Environ. Health Perspect.*, 107(4):297.

[2] Nordenvall A. S., Frisén L., Nordenström A., et al. (2014) A Population-Based Nationwide Study of Hypospadias in Sweden, 1973–2009: Incidence and Risk Factors. *J. Urol.,* 191(3):783-9.

[3] Tourchi A., Hoebeke P. (2013) Long-term outcome of male genital reconstruction in childhood. *J. Ped. Urol.*, 9(6 pt B):980-9.

[4] Nassar N., Bower C., Barker A. (2007) Increasing prevalence of hypospadias in Western Australia, 1980–2000. *Arch. Dis. Child.,* 92(7): 580-4.

[5] Canon S., Mosley B., Chipollini J., et al. (2012) Epidemiological Assessment of Hypospadias by Degree of Severity. *J. Urol.,* 188(6): 2362-6.

[6] Parker S. E., Mai C. T., Canfield M. A., et al. (2010) Updated national birth prevalence estimates for selected birth defects in the United States,

2004–2006. *Birth Defects Res., Part A.: Clin. Mol. Teratol.,* 88(12): 1008-16.

[7] Gatti J., Kirsch A., Troyer W., et al. (2001) Increased incidence of hypospadias in small-for-gestational age infants in a neonatal intensive-care unit. *BJU Int.*, 87(6):548-50.

[8] Huisma F., Thomas M., Armstrong L. (2013) Severe hypospadias and its association with maternal-placental factors. *Am. J. Med. Genet.,* Part A. 161?(9):2183-7.

[9] Yinon Y., Proctor L. K., Kelly E. N., et al. (2010) Hypospadias in males with intrauterine growth restriction due to placental insufficiency: the placental role in the embryogenesis of male external genitalia. *Am. J. Med. Genet.,* Part A. 152(1):75-83.

[10] Porter M. P., Faizan M. K., Grady R. W., Mueller B. A. (2005) Hypospadias in Washington State: maternal risk factors and prevalence trends. *Pediatrics,* 115(4):e495-e9.

[11] Kalfa N., Philibert P., Baskin L., Sultan C. Hypospadias: interactions between environment and genetics. *Molecular and Cellular Endocrinology,* 2011; 335(2):89 95.

[12] Rooij I. A., Zanden L. F., Brouwers M. M., et al. (2013) Risk factors for different phenotypes of hypospadias: results from a Dutch case–control study. *BJU Int.*, 112(1):121-8.

[13] Fujimoto T., Suwa T., Kabe K., et al. (2008) Placental insufficiency in early gestation is associated with hypospadias. *J. Pediatr. Surg.,* 43(2): 358-61.

[14] Brouwers M. M., Feitz W. F., Roelofs L. A.,et al. (2007) Risk factors for hypospadias. *Eur. J. Pediatr.,* 166(7):671-8.

[15] Hjartaker A., Ballard-Barbash R., Veierød M. B., et al. (2007) 17-beta-Estradiol in relation to age at menarche and adult obesity in premenopausal women. *Hum. Reprod.,* 23(4):919-27.

[16] Pierre Mouriquand. (2007) Dialogues in Pediatric Urology. *J. Ped. Urol.,* 28.

[17] Carmichael S. L., Shaw G. M., Nelson V., et al. (2003) Hypospadias in California: trends and descriptive epidemiology. *Epidemiology,* 14(6):701-6.

[18] Carlson W. H., Kisely S. R., MacLellan D. L. (2009) Maternal and fetal risk factors associated with severity of hypospadias: a comparison of mild and severe cases. *J. Ped. Urol.,* 5(4):283-6.

[19] Pierik F. H., Burdorf A., Deddens J. A., et al. (2004) Maternal and paternal risk factors for cryptorchidism and hypospadias: a case–control study in newborn boys. *Environ. Health Perspect.,* 112(15):1570.

[20] Main K. M., Skakkebæk N. E., Virtanen H. E., et al. (2010) Genital anomalies in boys and the environment. *Best Prac. Res. Clin. Endocrinol. Metab.,* 24(2):279-89.

[21] Klip H., Verloop J., van Gool J. D., et al. (2002) . Hypospadias in sons of women exposed to diethylstilbestrol in utero: a cohort study. *Lancet,* 359 (9312):1102-7.

[22] Bang J. K., Lyu S. W., Choi J., et al. (2013). Does infertility treatment increase male reproductive tract disorder? *Urology,* 81(3):644-8.

[23] Silver R. I., Rodriguez R., Chang T. S.,et al. (1999). In vitro fertilization is associated with an increased risk of hypospadias. *J. Urol.,* 161(6): 1954-7.

[24] Olson C. K., Keppler-Noreuil K. M., Romitti P. A., et al. (2005) In vitro fertilization is associated with an increase in major birth defects. *Fertility Steril.,* 84(5):1308-15.

[25] Baskin L. S., Himes K., Colborn T. (2001) Hypospadias and endocrine disruption: is there a connection? *Environ. Health Perspect.,* 109(11): 1175.

[26] Colborn T., vom Saal F. S., Soto A. M. (1993) Developmental effects of endocrine-disrupting chemicals in wildlife and humans. *Environ. Health Perspect.*, 101(5):378.

[27] Rocheleau C. M., Romitti P. A., Dennis L. K. (2009) Pesticides and hypospadias: a meta-analysis. *J. Ped. Urol.*, 5(1):17-24.

[28] Rocheleau C. M., Romitti P. A., Sanderson W. T., et al. (2011) Maternal occupational pesticide exposure and risk of hypospadias in the national birth defects prevention study. *Birth Defects Res. Part A: Clin. Mol. Teratol.,* 91(11):927-36.

[29] Li M., Qiu L., Zhang Y., et al. (2013) Dose-related effect by maternal exposure to di-(2-ethylhexyl) phthalate plasticizer on inducing hypospadiac male rats. *Environ. Toxicol. Pharmacol.*, 35(1):55-60.

[30] Klinefelter G. R., Laskey J. W., Winnik W. M., et al. (2012) Novel molecular targets associated with testicular dysgenesis induced by gestational exposure to diethylhexyl phthalate in the rat: a role for estradiol. *Reprod.,* 144(6):747-61.

[31] Van der Zanden L., van Rooij I., Feitz W., et al. (2012) Aetiology of hypospadias: a systematic review of genes and environment. *Hum. Reprod. Update,* 18(3):260-83.

[32] Choi H., Kim J., Im Y., et al. (2012) The association between some endocrine disruptors and hypospadias in biological samples. *J. Environ. Sci. Health,* Part A. 47(13):2173-9.

[33] Carmichael S. L., Cogswell M. E., Ma C., et al. (2013) Hypospadias and Maternal Intake of Phytoestrogens. *Am. J. Epidemiol.*, 178(3): 434-40.

[34] Schnack T. H., Poulsen G., Myrup C., et al. (2010) Familial coaggregation of cryptorchidism, hypospadias, and testicular germ cell cancer: a nationwide cohort study. *J. Natl. Cancer Inst.,* 102 (3):187-92.

[35] Whiteford M. (2004) Genetic aspects of hypospadias. *Hypospadias Surg.*, 59-61.

[36] Sharpe R. M. (2003) The 'oestrogen hypothesis'–where do we stand now? 1. *Int. J. Androl.,* 26(1):2-15.

[37] Norgil Damgaard I., Maria Main K., Toppari J., et al. (2002). Impact of exposure to endocrine disrupters< i> inutero</i> and in childhood on adult reproduction. *Best Prac. Res. Clin. Endocrinol. Metab.,* 16 (2): 289-309.

[38] Carmichael S. L., Ma C., Feldkamp M. L., et al. (2012) Nutritional factors and hypospadias risks. *Paediatr. Perinat. Epidemiol.*, 26(4): 353-60.

[39] North K., Golding J. A maternal vegetarian diet in pregnancy is associated with hypospadias. *BJU international.,* 2000;85(1):107-13.

[40] Giannandrea F. (2009) Correlation analysis of cocoa consumption data with worldwide incidence rates of testicular cancer and hypospadias. *Int. J. Environ. Res. Public Health*, 6(2):568-78.

[41] Brouwers M. M., Van Der Zanden L. F., De Gier R. P., et al. (2010) Hypospadias: risk factor patterns and different phenotypes. *BJU Int.,* 105(2):254-62.

[42] Akre O., Boyd H. A., Ahlgren M., et al. (2008) Maternal and gestational risk factors for hypospadias. *Environ. Health Perspect.,* 116(8):1071.

[43] Vajda F. J., O'Brien T. J., Graham J. E., et al. (2013) Dose dependence of fetal malformations associated with valproate. *Neurology,* 81(11): 999-1003.

[44] Yakoob M. Y., Bateman B. T., Ho E., et al. (2013) The Risk of Congenital Malformations Associated With Exposure to β-Blockers Early in Pregnancy A Meta-Analysis. *Hypertension,* 62(2):375-81.

[45] Quinonez S. C., Park J. M., Rabah R., et al. (2013) 9p partial monosomy and disorders of sex development: Review and postulation of a pathogenetic mechanism. *Am. J. Med. Genet., Part A.* 161(8):1882-96.

[46] Vottero A., Minari R., Viani I., et al.(2011) Evidence for epigenetic abnormalities of the androgen receptor gene in foreskin from children with hypospadias. *J. Clin. Endocrinol. Metab.,* 96(12):E1953-E62.

[47] Parada-Bustamante A., Lardone M. C., Madariaga M., et al. (2012) Androgen receptor CAG and GGN polymorphisms in boys with isolated hypospadias. *J. Ped. Endocrinol. Metab.*, 25(1-2):157-62.

[48] Wang Y., Li Q., Xu J., et al. (2004) Mutation analysis of five candidate genes in Chinese patients with hypospadias. *Eur. J. Hum. Genet.,* 12(9): 706-12.

[49] Palazzolo I., Gliozzi A., Rusmini P., et al. (2008) The role of the polyglutamine tract in androgen receptor. *J. Steroid. Biochem. Mol. Biol.,* 108(3):245-53.

[50] Crabbe P., Bogaert V., De Bacquer D., et al. (2007) Part of the interindividual variation in serum testosterone levels in healthy men reflects differences in androgen sensitivity and feedback set point: contribution of the androgen receptor polyglutamine tract polymorphism. *J. Clin. Endocrinol. Metab.,* 92(9):3604-10.

[51] Radpour R., Rezaee M., Tavasoly A., et al. (2007) Association of long polyglycine tracts (GGN repeats) in exon 1 of the androgen receptor gene with cryptorchidism and penile hypospadias in Iranian patients. *J. Androl.*, 28(1):164-9.

[52] Aschim E. L., Nordenskjöld A., Giwercman A., et al. (2004) Linkage between cryptorchidism, hypospadias, and GGN repeat length in the androgen receptor gene. *J. Clin. Endocrinol. Metab.*, 89(10):5105-9.

[53] Rusmini P., Bolzoni E., Crippa V., et al. (2010) Proteasomal and autophagic degradative activities in spinal and bulbar muscular atrophy. *Neurobiol. Dis.,* 40(2):361-9.

[54] Choudhry S., Deshpande A., Qiao L., et al. (2012) Genome-wide DNA Methylation Profiling of CpG Islands in Hypospadias. *J. Urol.,* 188(4 suppl.):1450-5.

[55] Lottrup G., Jørgensen A., Nielsen J. E., et al. (2013) Identification of a novel androgen receptor mutation in a family with multiple components compatible with the testicular dysgenesis syndrome. *J. Clin. Endocrinol. Metab.,* 98(6):2223-9.

[56] Codner E. O. C., Iniguez G., Boric M. A., et al. (2004) Molecular study of the 3 beta-hydroxysteroid dehydrogenase gene type II in patients with hypospadias. *J. Clin. Endocrinol. Metab.,* 89.

[57] Rey R. A., Codner E., Iñíguez G., et al. (2005) Low risk of impaired testicular Sertoli and Leydig cell functions in boys with isolated hypospadias. *J. Clin. Endocrinol. Metabolism,* 90(11):6035-40.
[58] Carmichael S. L., Mohammed N., Ma C., et al. (2013) Diacylglycerol Kinase K Variants Impact Hypospadias in a California Study Population. *J. Urol.,* 189(1):305-11.
[59] van der Zanden L. F., van Rooij I. A., Feitz W. F., et al. (2010) Common variants in DGKK are strongly associated with risk of hypospadias. *Nat. Genet.,* 43(1):48-50.
[60] Imai S. K. M., Yasuda S. et al. (2005) Identification and characterization of a novel human type II diacylglycerol kinase, DGK kappa. *J. Biol. Chem.*, 280:39870.
[61] McMahon A. P., Aronow B. J., Davidson D. R., et al. (2008) GUDMAP: the genitourinary developmental molecular anatomy project. *J. Am. Soci. Nephrol.*, 19(4):667-71.
[62] Zanden L., Galesloot T., Feitz W., et al. 2012 Exploration of gene-environment interactions, maternal effects and parent of origin effects in the etiology of hypospadias. *J. Urol.*, 188(6) 2351 60.
[63] Beleza-Meireles A., Töhönen V., Söderhäll C., et al. (2008) Activating transcription factor 3: a hormone responsive gene in the etiology of hypospadias. *Eur. J. Endocrinol.,* 158(5):729-39.
[64] Wang M. H., Baskin L. S. (2008) Endocrine disruptors, genital development, and hypospadias. *J. Andrology,* 29(5):499-505.
[65] Wang Z., Liu B. C., Lin G. T., et al. (2007) Up-regulation of estrogen responsive genes in hypospadias: microarray analysis. *J. Urol.* 177(5): 1939-46.
[66] Barlow N. J., Phillips S. L., Wallace D. G., et al. (2003) Quantitative changes in gene expression in fetal rat testes following exposure to di (n-butyl) phthalate. *Toxicol. Sci.*, 73(2):431-41.
[67] Irizarry R. A., Ladd-Acosta C., Wen B., et al. (2009) The human colon cancer methylome shows similar hypo-and hypermethylation at conserved tissue-specific CpG island shores. *Nat. Genet.,* 41(2):178-86.
[68] Li M., Qiu L., Lin T., et al. (2013) c-Jun N-Terminal Kinase is Upregulated in Patients With Hypospadias. *Urology,* 81(1):178-83.
[69] Ogata T., Sano S., Nagata E., Kato F., Fukami M., editors. MAMLD1 and 46, XY Disorders of Sex Development. Seminars in reproductive medicine; 2012: Thieme Medical Publishers.

[70] El-Khairi R., Achermann J. C., editors. Steroidogenic Factor-1 and Human Disease. Seminars in reproductive medicine; 2012: Thieme Medical Publishers.

[71] Carmichael S., Witte J., Ma C., (2014) Hypospadias and variants in genes related to sex hormone biosynthesis and metabolism. *Andrology,* 2(1):130-7.

[72] Latronico A. C. A. I. (2012) Inactivating mutations of the human luteinizing hormone receptor in both sexes. *Semin. Reprod. Med.,* 30(5): 382-6.

[73] Kojima Y., Kohri K., Hayashi Y. (2010) Genetic pathway of external genitalia formation and molecular etiology of hypospadias. *J. Ped. Urol.,* 6(4):346-54.

[74] Sajjad Y. (2010) Development of the genital ducts and external genitalia in the early human embryo. *J. Obs. Gyn. Res.,* 36(5):929-37.

[75] Lee D. K., Chang C. (2003) Molecular communication between androgen receptor and general transcription machinery. *J. Steroid. Biochem. Mol. Biol.*, 84(1):41-9.

[76] Pfeifer K. (2000) Mechanisms of genomic imprinting. *Am. J. Hum. Genet.,* 67(4):777-87.

[77] Qin X.-Y., Kojima Y., Mizuno K., et al.(2012) Association of variants in genes involved in environmental chemical metabolism and risk of cryptorchidism and hypospadias. *J. Hum. Genet.,* 57(7):434-41.

[78] Virtanen H. E., Adamsson A. (2012) Cryptorchidism and endocrine disrupting chemicals. *Mol. Cell. Endocrinol.*, 355(2):208-20.

[79] Fukami M. (2012) A Commentary on Association of variants in genes involved in environmental chemical metabolism and risk of cryptorchidism and hypospadias. *J. Hum. Genet.*, 57(7):405-6.

[80] Meijer W. M., de Jong-Van den Berg L., van den Berg M. D., et al. (2006) Clomiphene and hypospadias on a detailed level: signal or chance? *Birth Defects Res. Part A: Clin. Mol. Teratol.,* 76(4):249-52.

In: Hypospadias
Editor: Daniel H. Preston
ISBN: 978-1-63482-023-3

Chapter 3

Current State of Tissue Engineering for Repair of Congenital Hypospadias

Jessica H. Hannick[1,*] ***and Arun K. Sharma***[2]

[1]Department of Urology, Loyola University Medical Center, Maywood, IL, US

[2]Ann & Robert H. Lurie Children's Hospital of Chicago, Division of Pediatric Urology, Chicago, IL, US

Northwestern University Feinberg School of Medicine, Department of Urology, Chicago, IL, US

Northwestern University, Simpson Querrey Institute for BioNanotechnology, Chicago, IL, US

Northwestern University Department of Biomedical Engineering, Evanston, IL, US

Abstract

In the past several decades, numerous advances in the field of tissue engineering have been made towards the management of hypospadias and associated urethral defects. Reliable products for clinical use still remain

* Corresponding author: jhannick@lumc.edu.

elusive, however. Hypospadias affects approximately 0.3% of live births with current practice favoring early repair. With the advances in surgical approaches to hypospadias repair, such as the tubularized-incised plate, mid-shaft and distal variants rarely require supplemental tissue. In more proximal and perineal urethral defects, and especially in the case of the hypospadias cripple, however, patients may lack adequate, healthy local tissue for definitive repair. Ongoing research into the use of acellular matrix grafts and cell-seeded matrix grafts have produced promising results in animal models. Unfortunately, these grafts can be plagued by graft loss, graft contracture, stricture formation, and fistulization. Extensive additional research remains to evaluate the long-term biosafety and efficacy of these materials and to determine a reproducible and cost-effective means for their use in clinical practice.

Introduction

Historical rates of hypospadias in live-births range from 1/125-1000, however epidemiologic evidence indicates that the incidence may be on the rise. Recent analyses of nationwide health registries of males born in Sweden from 1973-2009 indicated rates of 4.5 per 1,000 live-births till 1990 almost doubling to 8 per 1,000 live-births over the following ten years [1]. In their review of newborn males discharged from California hospitals from 1985-2006, however, Elliott et al. found that the rate of hypospadias was relatively constant, with a mean rate of 42 cases per 10,000 live male births [2].

Though surgical intervention is rarely urgently required, to minimize psychological trauma associated with repair, early intervention is typically recommended. The ultimate goal of surgery is to construct a penis with an appearance and function as close to normal as possible [3]. The three basic categories of hypospadias repair include tubularization of the urethral plate, substitution or reinforcement of the urethral plate with local flaps, or substitution of the urethral plate with exogenous grafts. The first of these comprises the most commonly utilized technique, however, occasionally patients will have significant isolated urethral length deficiency, a large urethral defect after release of chordee, or have undergone several prior failed urethral surgeries and now have fibrotic, poorly vascularized local tissues and therefore require graft urethroplasty. Similar scenarios are seen in the adult population in men with significant urethral length loss due to urethral stricture disease. Mirroring the treatment approach of urethral stricture repair, various grafts have been tested and applied in substitution or replacement urethroplasty for hypospadias repair.

First described by Humby in 1941, buccal mucosal grafts have become one of the most widely used graft tissues used in first-stage complicated urethroplasties and re-do urethroplasties for hypospadias and urethral strictures [4]. Their widespread acceptance has been attributed to their histologic properties and minimal morbidity of harvesting. Buccal mucosal grafts exhibit a thin lamina propria layer which has been theorized to aid in rapid neovascularization and graft take. Grafts are either harvested from the inner lips or cheek and can be performed concomitantly with implantation. Potential morbidity of buccal mucosal grafts includes post-operative pain, delayed return to general diet, swelling, and peri-oral numbness [5]. Specifically in harvests from the cheek, attention must be paid to avoid Stensen's duct, or alteration in salivary gland function may occur.

Though buccal mucosa offers clinicians a readily available autologous source of graft material, it is a finite material in each patient and does not come without morbidity and risk. As a result, in the past several decades, researchers have sought to generate alternative sources of tissue for urethral grafting.

Basic Principles of Tissue Engineering

The ideal urethral substitute must be one that incorporates well into the surrounding milieu after implantation, does not experience any contraction, fibrosis, immune rejection, or exaggerated inflammatory response, is impermeable, inexpensive, and is easily handled without tear or fracture [6]. Construction of this graft fundamentally relies on a scaffold with or without cells, referred to respectively as acellular and cellular grafts. The scaffold serves to mimic the function of native extracellular matrix (ECM) by providing a physical support as well as bioactive factors. With cellular grafts, a cell-adhesion substrate is often required for cells to anchor to the scaffold. Therefore, the cells are often loaded with cell-adhesion peptides and growth factors to modulate their adherence to the graft [7]. Scaffolds fall into three categories, synthetic, naturally derived materials, and acellular tissue matrices. Whereas synthetic scaffolds can be manufactured in large and reliably reproducible volumes with consistent properties, they are foreign to native tissues and pose a risk of rejection unlike naturally derived materials and acellular tissue matrices.

Graft Scaffold Materials

Synthetic materials currently used as scaffolds are the biodegradable polymers poly(glycolic acid) (PGA), poly(lactic acid) (PLA), and poly(lactic acid-co-glycolic acid) (PLGA) [6, 7]. These materials can be manufactured in variable, yet consistent three-dimensional structures at a relatively low cost without the requirement of harvesting from a donor. The manufacturer can also vary the permeability as well as other mechanical properties of the synthetic scaffold.

Once implanted, these materials are naturally hydrolyzed and then cleared through metabolic pathways [8-10]. Aside from the potential risk of foreign body rejection, these scaffolds also lack natural cell-signaling factors that guide cell implantation and fate if cell-seeding is desired.

As an abundantly available resource native to the extracellular environment, collagen can be extracted from either human or animal tissues for use as a scaffold. Collagen is approved by the U.S Food and Drug Administration and exhibits minimal antigenic responses when implanted [11]. Fossum and Nordenskjöld used a collagen matrix scaffold derived from their patients' own skin which was de-epithelialized to yield an acellular dermis [12]. This approach, however, necessitates a skin grafting procedure with potential graft site complications such as poor cosmesis, infection, and/or pain.

Small intestinal submucosa (SIS) and acellular bladder matrix (ABM) have been used as alternative biological acellular matrices [6, 7]. These also possess many functional and mechanical properties similar to native ECM. As these tissues slowly degrade, they are replaced by newly modeled ECM proteins secreted by either nearby cells or ingrowing cells, in the case of cellular grafts. While these scaffolds exhibit minimal immune reactions or rejection, their composition may be largely variable, and their acquisition costly. When acquired from non-human subjects, they also carry the potential for disease transmission, immune reactions, or rejection [7].

Clinical History of Acellular Grafts

Acellular grafts have been in clinical use for several years. They may only be used when nearby healthy urethral tissues are present, however, as the acellular graft is meant to serve as a scaffold for surrounding urothelial and connective tissue to grow over, bridging the gap between deficient areas. As a result, these are not appropriate options for the management of severe proximal or perineal hypospadias, where the gap between healthy tissues is too great, or in the case of the hypospadias cripple, where nearby tissues are fibrotic and lack adequate vascularity [6].

In 1999, Chen et al. applied the use of a bladder collagen matrix to an animal urethroplasty model [13]. A 1x0.7cm ventral urethral defect was created in 10 rabbits. Acellular collagen matrix was obtained from porcine bladder submucosa and placed on the defects in an onlay approach. The rabbits were followed with pre- and post-operative retrograde urethrogram (RUG) at 0.5, 1, 2, 3, and 6 months after graft urethroplasty. A cohort of animals was sacrificed at each of those time points. Post-implantation RUGs in all of the animals demonstrated adequate caliber urethras with no radiographic evidence of stricture disease. On gross inspection, all of the grafted urethras appeared to have normal tissue with no fibrosis. Whereas pre-op histologic examination confirmed that the collagen grafts were acellular, post-op examination revealed angiogenesis and a complete layer of transitional cell epithelium at 2 weeks and then maintained throughout, which was confirmed on immunohistochemistry.

Atala et al. reported in the same year on their use of collagen matrix into human hypospadias repair in four patients with a history of failed hypospadias repairs (3 penoscrotal and 1 scrotal) [14]. Collagen matrix grafts were obtained from cadaveric donor bladder submucosa. The patient's neourethral lengths ranged 5-15cm. The urethral plates were not excised, and the grafts were incorporated in an onlay fashion. Patients underwent RUG and cystoscopy with biopsy at 1 year following repair. One patient, the 20 year old who required a 15cm neourethra developed a 2cm penile fistula in the subglanular region, which was detected at 6 wks post-op and repaired with standard techniques. At 1 year, follow-up RUGs in all patients were patent with biopsies revealing urethral stratified epithelium.

Expanding on the urethral stricture literature, in 2003 the Atala group performed urethral reconstruction with collagen matrix via onlay repair in 28 adult patients with urethral stricture [15]. Donor human cadaveric bladder submucosa was used as the collagen matrix graft after excising the diseased urethral plate to create neourethras ranging from 1.5-16cm. Patients were evaluated post-operatively with RUG and uroflowmetry and cystoscopy at 4 mos post-operatively with mean follow-up 37 months (range 36-48 months). Success incorporated visualization of an adequate caliber urethra on RUG. Twenty-four of the twenty-eight repairs were deemed successful. The remaining four patients required direct vision internal urethrotomy (DVIU) with no need for subsequent procedures. One patient experienced a subcoronal fistula post-operatively which resolved spontaneously by 1 year post-op.

In 2008, the Atala group compared their results of urethroplasty with acellular collagen matrices to those with buccal mucosal grafts [16]. Thirty adult patients with complex urethral strictures ranging in length from 2-18cm underwent urethroplasty, five with human acellular cadaveric donor bladder matrix and six with buccal mucosa. The etiologies of the strictures were varied, with two strictures resulting from failed previous hypospadias repairs. In patients with strictured segments greater than 5cm in length or associated with significant fibrosis, a Russell's procedure was performed to shorten the length of the required graft and remove fibrosis. Patients were divided into those with 0-1 previous repairs or 2 or more previous repairs. Postoperatively, patients were evaluated via uroflowmetry and ascending and voiding urethrography for a mean follow-up 25 months. Success was defined as maintenance of a normal voiding pattern with a steady stream without weakening over time and no further need for intervention. In the first group, 10/10 (100%) of buccal grafts were successful, and 8/9 (89%) of the acellular matrix grafts were successful. In the second group, those patients with a history of two or more previous repairs, 5/5 (100%) of buccal grafts were successful, whereas only 2/6 (33%) of acellular matrix grafts were successful. Those patients that failed developed strictures requiring additional procedures. The writers noted that graft success was directly linked to the quality of urethral bed, which is inherently important to the graft, as new grafts require adequate neovascularization to survive. They concluded that acellular collagen matrices are a viable option in patients with healthy urethral plates and minimal spongiofibrosis as this alternate material avoids the need for tissue harvest.

Turning to the SIS literature, in 2006 Donkov et al. used SIS in nine men with urethral strictures ranging in length from 4-6cm [17]. The study subjects all underwent preoperative evaluation with RUG and uroflowmetry. During the repair, their strictures were incised dorsally, and then a four-layered SIS graft, 4mm larger than the dorsal urethral site, was laid over the dorsally incised area. The inner surface of the patch was gently fenestrated with a scalpel, the mucosa was sutured 2-3mm inwards from margin, and then the spongiosum was sutured to the margins. One patient restrictured at 6 months post-operatively, however, he was found to have E. coli urethritis at that time. Uroflowmetry ranged 20-22 mL/s from 10-16 mL/s pre-operatively. Six of the patients had post-void dribbling, however none found it bothersome. Cystoscopy at 3 months demonstrated gross complete urothelial regeneration. Some of the patients had issues with erectile dysfunction post-operatively, but in all patients this either resolved or was medically managed. A qualitative questionnaire given to the study participants revealed that all preferred to have tissue used in repair that had not been taken from them.

In a similar study, fifty men with anterior urethral strictures ranging in length from 4-14cm underwent urethroplasty with porcine SIS-collagen based matrix [18]. Patients were evaluated with pre- and post-operative voiding diaries, antegrade and retrograde urethrograms, and cystoscopy. Success was measured by the absence of a stricture on urethrography. The strictures were incised and an SIS graft was placed via dorsal onlay. With a mean follow-up of 31.2 months, 10/50 patients experienced graft failure within 6 months and required further therapy. Following these interventions, however, there were no subsequent failures. Of note, none of the patients experienced complications such as fistula, wound infection, urinary tract infection, or graft rejection.

Mirroring Donkov's study population and outcomes, in 2012 Palminteri et al. studied 25 men with bulbar urethral strictures ranging in size from 1.5-6cm [19]. In all patients, after the stricture was incised, the fibrotic urethral tissues were partially excised while preserving the remaining urethral plate. The patients then underwent patch graft with graft sizes ranging 4-7cm, using 4-layer SIS placed dorsally or ventrally or dorsally and ventrally in an on-lay patch fashion. The repair was deemed a failure if post-operative instrumentation was required, i.e. urethral dilation. With a mean follow-up of 71 months, six failures (24%) were noted. There were no postoperative complications directly related to the graft material (i.e. infection or graft rejection). When the patients were subcategorized based on stricture length, the failure rate for strictures <4cm was 14%, and for strictures > 4cm it was 100%.

The authors concluded that "the use of SIS as graft material should not be the first choice but represents an alternative option for patients with bulbar strictures that are not long and who refuse the harvesting or are not ideal candidates for buccal mucosa or penile skin grafts."

Seeking to see how acellular grafts might function if tubularized, Dorin et al. investigated the maximal length of unseeded tubularized graft that could be used to achieve new urothelial growth before fibrosis developed [20]. Tubularized urethroplasties were performed in 12 male rabbits using acellular matrices of bladder submucosa with varying lengths (0.5, 1, 2, and 3 cm). Following implantation, serial urethrography was performed at 1, 3, and 4 weeks. RUG was normal for the 0.5cm group at all time points, however, strictures were noted in the 1, 2, and 3 cm graft groups by 4 weeks. Graft harvest and staining at 1, 3, and 4 week time-points demonstrated ingrowth of urothelium from the anastomotic sites by 1 week. By 4 weeks, the 0.5cm graft had a normal transitional layer surrounded by a muscle layer within the wall of the lumen. In the 1, 2, and 3cm groups, however, there was only ingrowth at the anastomotic edges with collagen deposition and fibrosis towards the center of the grafts by 2 weeks and extensive fibrosis throughout the grafts at 4 weeks. From these findings, the authors concluded that the maximal defect distance suitable for a tubularized acellular graft is 0.5cm with otherwise healthy surrounding tissue.

Graft Cells

Two basic populations of cells exist for use in tissue engineering of the urethra: progenitor cells and stem cells. Because of their similarities between the scaffold and cells used, much of the knowledge derived from experience with constructing tissue engineered bladders has been translated into the realm of urethral reconstruction.

Progenitor cells originate within many organs, but have limited reproductive capacity and for their specific cell type only [6, 7]. They are responsible for tissue maintenance during the normal course of cell turn-over, death, and regeneration. Progenitor cells utilize the principle of extracting autologous cells from an individual, culturing and expanding them, and then implanting them into a target site to ultimately be incorporated into native tissues. Among epithelial cell types, autologous urothelial, epidermal, and oral keratinocytes have been used in tissue engineering. Autologous urothelial cells traditionally have been extracted from the bladder via bladder biopsy, however, due to the invasiveness of this approach, techniques have been developed to isolate these cells either from bladder washes or voided urine [21, 22]. Epidermal cells are readily available in the uncircumcised male, but in the circumcised male or if using buccal mucosa, the patient is subjected to the morbidity of a graft harvest. Consideration must be given to the use of autologous urothelial cells in patients with dysfunctional bladders, however, as these cells may be at risk for similar disease processes such as fibrosis, poor elasticity, and overall subpar functionality.

In contrast to progenitor cells, stem cells are undifferentiated cells capable of self-renewal that can differentiate into mature non-reproductive cells [6, 7]. These can be obtained from embryos, however, due to ethical considerations they are more frequently obtained from adult bone marrow, adipose tissue, and urine. Retrieving stem cells from bone marrow is often a painful process for the donor and yields a low proportion of mesenchymal stem cells (MSCs) which require ex-vivo expansion [23]. The most abundant and accessible of these sources is adipose tissue, however, a population of urine-derived cells has been identified as well [6]. The use of stem cells can be of particular interest when engineered grafts are indicated in patients whose urothelial progenitor cells may be otherwise diseased or malignant, such as patients with a history of a neurogenic bladder, pelvic radiation, or bladder malignancy.

Another issue associated with the use of stem cells has been malignancy. Aside from the previously mentioned ethical concerns, embryonic stem cells have been known to proliferate and differentiate into teratomas when implanted into immune-suppressed mice [24, 25]. Conflicting reports exist regarding the malignant potential of adult MSCs. Bernardo et al. demonstrated long-term in-vitro culture of bone marrow-derived MSCs yielded no malignant transformation [26]. Røsland et al., however, observed rapid cell proliferation and spontaneous malignant transformation, which manifested as numerous pulmonary malignant deposits after injection into immune-suppressed mice [27]. Similar results were confirmed by Rubio el al using adipose tissue-derived MSCs [28].

Clinical History of Cellular Grafts

Cell-seeded grafts were developed for use either as tubularized urethral grafts to replace large segments of urethra or in patients where local urethral tissue is both deficient and inadequate to support de novo tissue regeneration.

Attempting to merge prior experience from buccal mucosal grafting with the use of cell-seeded grafts, Bhargava et al.l studied five patients with urethral stricture secondary to lichen sclerosis who underwent urethroplasty with autologous tissue-engineered buccal mucosal grafts [29]. Buccal mucosa biopsies (0.5cm) were obtained under local anesthetic. These were processed and the dermis separated from keratinocytes. The cells were then cultured and expanded and three pieces of either 3x5cm or 3x10cm grafts were cultured for each patient. Biopsies of the grafts were taken to confirm they were morphologically similar to buccal mucosa. Urethroplasty was then performed either as a two-stage (insufficient graft size in 1 patient, 1 patient had 11cm graft placed for penobulbar stricture, other patient not discussed) or a one-stage procedure (2 patients). The initial graft take was 100%, though one patient later required complete graft excision and another patient required partial graft excision due to fibrosis and hyperproliferation of tissue. The remaining patients required either DVIU or intermittent meatal dilations for strictures. These results were not considered ideal, especially since the patients required a buccal mucosa biopsy, and as a result, this approach didn't save them much time or the potential morbidity of standard buccal mucosal graft, nor were the surgical outcomes markedly better.

Subsequent studies have attempted to use urothelial cells to seed acellular grafts. Filippo et al. created 1cm tubularized acellular collagen matrices from decellularized porcine bladder tissue [30]. These matrices were then seeded with bladder cells from ten rabbits, obtained via open bladder biopsy. A 1cm urethral segment was excised in 24 rabbits. Urethroplasty was then performed in 12 rabbits with cell-seeded tubularized collagen matrix and in 12 rabbits with unseeded tubularized collagen matrix. Urethrography was performed pre-operatively and at 1, 2, 3, and 6 months post-operatively. The urethras were then harvested and examined histologically. Urethrography in seeded grafts demonstrated wide caliber at all time points, whereas in unseeded grafts, there were strictures and graft collapse at all time points. Seeded grafts had transitional cell layer with muscle fibers by 1 month and increasing organization of muscle as time progressed. Unseeded grafts also demonstrated transitional epithelium, but minimal unorganized muscle bundles were seen, and mostly at anastomotic sites only. Organ bath studies demonstrated seeded grafts were also capable of contraction similar to that of the normal urethra when stimulated by cholinergic and muscarinic receptor agonists. These promising results meant that seeded grafts might be an alternative option for urethral substitution. An open bladder biopsy procedure was used, however, thus reducing any benefit over buccal mucosal graft harvesting.

Seeking to use a more readily available source of cells, though still not obviating the need for cell harvest, Fu harvested rabbit foreskin epidermal cells from 9 rabbits [31]. The epidermal cells were expanded in vitro and seeded onto an acellular collagen matrix created from rabbit bladder submucosa. A 1.5cm penile urethral defect was created in 18 male rabbits. Urethroplasty was performed with tubularized seeded collagen matrix (9 rabbits) or unseeded collagen matrix (9 rabbits). Urethrography was performed at 1, 2, and 6 months after grafting and demonstrated strictures at various time points in the unseeded group, whereas the seeded group had wide caliber urethras throughout at all time points. Histology in the unseeded control group at 1 month revealed a single layer of epithelial cells with disorganized muscle fibers in the submucosa and at two and six months there were transitional cell layers surrounded by disorganized muscle fibers. In the seeded group, histology at 1 month revealed a single-layer structure, whereas at two and six months there were several layers of epidermal cells with abundant submucosal vessels. At 6 months, there was a distinct margin between graft epidermal cells and host epithelial cells in the seeded graft group. Immunofluorescence over the course of study demonstrated a transition from grafted cells to ingrowth of new cells, and the grafted cells were phased out. This study clearly demonstrated the superiority of tissue regeneration in seeded versus unseeded collagen matrix grafts in the rabbit urethroplasty model.

Expanding on Fu's 2007 study, Orabi et al. translated similar methods into a canine preclinical model [32]. Autologous bladder and epithelial smooth muscle cells were harvested via an open 2cm x 2cm bladder biopsy from fifteen dogs. The cells were then expanded and seeded onto 6 cm long tubularized collagen-based matrices. A 6cm length of urethra was resected just distal to membranous urethra in 21 dogs and then concurrently replaced with either cell seeded graft (15 dogs) or unseeded collagen matrix (6 dogs). CT urethrograms and 3D scans were performed pre-operatively and at 1, 3, 6, and 12 months post-operatively. Urethrograms of the seeded grafts had no stricturing at all time points, whereas unseeded grafts demonstrated stricture formation within first 3 months. Urine leak was noted in all six acellular grafts, after removal of the urethral stent, and thought to be secondary to urethrocutaneous fistula development at the graft anastomotic sites. Gross examination of the seeded grafts appeared like that of normal, non-fibrotic urothelium. Histologic examination of the seeded grafts revealed epithelial cell growth with circumferential muscle cell fibers with increasing organization and bulk over time, whereas in the unseeded group there was an epithelial layer, dense fibrosis, and scant muscle cells observed. The positive results seen in the seeded graft group built upon the prior favorable studies, yet still did not exclude the requirement for an invasive procedure to obtain graft cells.

Given the positive precedent set for cell-seeded graft repairs, the animal model studies were then translated into a clinical human study. As in prior studies, an open suprapubic bladder biopsy (1x1cm) was taken from 5 male study subjects with a history of traumatic urethral strictures [33]. The bladder cells were grown for 3-6 weeks to obtain adequate cell numbers and then seeded onto a tubularized polyglycolide/polylactide biodegradable mesh scaffold with epithelial cells on the inner surface and muscle cells on the outer surface. RUG, voiding cystourethrogram (VCUG), and urethroscopy were performed pre-operatively, and then all five patients underwent urethroplasty with the graft composites. Patients were assessed post-operatively with a history, International Continence Society (ICS) questionnaire, urinalysis, RUG, cystoscopy, and uroflowmetry at 3, 6, 12, 24, 36, 48, 60, and 72 months after surgery. Post-operative median end max flow rate was 27.1 ml/s (range 16-28), and serial RUGs and cystoscopies demonstrated widely patent urethras in all patients. Serial graft biopsies performed endoscopically at 3, 6, 12, and 36 months demonstrated normal appearing tissues by 3 months post-urethroplasty. No fistulae or urinary tract infections were observed post-operatively. Patients were satisfied and reported no urinary symptoms. One patient developed narrowing at the anastomotic site 4 weeks post-operatively, which was incised with no subsequent issues. One patient with a history of traumatic pelvic disruption ultimately needed a sling for daytime stress urinary incontinence, however aside from this, all patients were considered continent post-urethroplasty.

In 2007, Fossum et al. utilized a similar technique for the treatment of 6 male patients with scrotal or perineal hypospadius and severe chordee [34]. The patients underwent a two-stage procedure; first with repair of chordee and bladder lavage for bladder cells, and 6 months later a definitive urethroplasty. The neourethras were created from an on-lay graft of cultured lavaged bladder cells which were seeded on acellular dermis (either human donor or commercial purchased). Following urethroplasty, the patients were seen at 2-4 weeks, 6 months, 1 year and then annually. At each of these visits, voiding position, urinary flow and cosmesis were observed for a follow-up range of 3-5.5 yrs. Urethroscopy and biopsy were also performed in each patient at unspecified time points. Post-operatively, all 6 boys voided without straining via their neourethra and had no residual urine. Five boys voided with a bell-shaped curve. The sixth developed a stricture at his proximal anastomosis which was initially treated with multiple catheterizations, but ultimately required DVIU at 12 months after urethroplasty. This patient reported no subjective complaints at 2 years after DVIU. Two boys developed urethrocutaneous fistulae which were treated with no recurrence or further issues. The cosmetic appearance was reported as good and associated with high parental satisfaction in all cases. Biopsies of three neourethras demonstrated urothelial cells, whereas two others yielded squamous cells, and one patient's biopsies were too small to analyze.

Emerging Horizons within Tissue Engineering

Although they undergo a decellularization and sterilization process, acellular matrices are criticized for their retention of residual DNA from exogenous ECM, which may lead to recipient rejection after graft implantation [6]. The self-assembly method produces tissues entirely composed of differentiated cells obtained from the graft recipient, including ECM from recipient fibroblasts. These tissues are autologous, hence eliminating the potential for immunologic reaction to the graft. The process of self-assembly is as follows; biopsies from the patient (fibroblasts [F] from skin or oral mucosa, adipose-derived stromal cells from skin, and smooth muscle and fibroblast cells from the bladder) are obtained. The Fs are isolated and then seeded into a custom-built tissue anchoring device, where they are then cultured and expanded with specific media to stimulate ECM synthesis. For approximately 21 days the cells are cultured until ECM proteins self-assemble into a sheet. These sheets are mostly composed of organized collagen I and III, the proteins most commonly seen in native bladder tissues. Urothelial cells are then seeded onto these self-assembled sheets and ultimately yield multi-layered, differentiated urothelium.

Permeability and tensile testing has yielded results similar and occasionally superior to that of native urethral tissues [35, 36]. No tears were noted when the engineered tissue was sutured together. When sutured grafts were subjected to tensile testing, they did leak, however, not until an internal pressure of 40 mmHg. A self-assembled matrix constructed from human adipose-derived stromal cells had similar structural and mechanical properties to that of the F self-assembled matrix [37]. When seeded with urothelial cells, however, there was inadequate proliferation of functional urothelium, therefore it was determined that the addition of fibroblasts was required. Criticisms of the self-assembly approach are its time-consuming nature and the persistent requirement for tissue biopsy from the graft recipient.

Given the known difficulty of graft vascularization and resultant fibrosis if inadequate neo-angiogenesis occurs, Imbeault et al. evaluated the effect on vascular proliferation of adding endothelial cells to self-assembled matrices [38]. To build the grafts, human dermal fibroblasts from skin biopsies after breast reduction, human urothelial cells from cadaveric bladder biopsies, and human umbilical vein endothelial cells from healthy newborns were obtained. Fs were cultured in media and supplemented with ascorbic acid to form a sheet, as previously described. After 25 days, endothelial cells were seeded onto the sheets for the study model (ET) and none for the standard tubular model (T). The sheets were tubularized two days later and then cultured for 21 days to fuse the cell layers. Each of the two model types were then intraluminally seeded with approximately 3 million urothelial cells and incubated in a bioreactor for one week. The completed grafts were then implanted subcutaneously, one into the right and one into the left dorsal muscles of male athymic nu/nu mice. At 7, 14, and 28 days after graft implantation, the mice were euthanized, and the grafts harvest and analyzed. Both the ET and T models exhibited pseudostratified urothelium luminally, robust ECM, and cohesion between layers. Biopsy prior to implantation showed capillaries in the ET model only, but they were observed in both models post-implantation, though more were seen in the ET model at 14 days and onward. T grafts had mouse RBCs and capillaries on the outer graft surface at 7 days and full graft thickness thereafter, but not as numerous as the ET models. In both models, capillaries increased in size as the time from implantation increased. As a result, this study demonstrated the importance of incorporating endothelial cells for more rapid and robust graft vascularization, an essential element for graft survival.

Conclusion

Within the past decade, significant advances have been made towards the development of an engineered tissue composite for use in hypospadias repair. In larger urethral defects, the evidence clearly supports seeded versus unseeded grafts, as these have demonstrated lower complication rates and better overall vascular, muscle, and urothelial tissue re-growth compared to unseeded grafts. The choice of optimal scaffold material remains unclear and requires more research. Unfortunately, researchers have not yet been able to develop a graft composite method that completely eliminates the need for tissue procurement and its potential morbidity. Graft cells also require a culture and expansion period to generate numbers adequate for scaffold seeding. Because of these reasons and the ongoing need for further human clinical studies, buccal mucosa grafting remains the mainstay of therapy for graft use in hypospadias repair. Future studies must attempt to minimize the morbidity of autologous cell harvest, reduce the interval between graft development and implantation, and evaluate cost-effectiveness, while maintaining parallel urothelial function and minimizing complications. Only then may an engineered urethral tissue have the opportunity to gain popularity in clinical practice.

References

[1] Nordenvall, AS; Frisén, L; Nordenström, A; Lichtenstein, P; Nordenskjöld, A. Population based nationwide study of hypospadias in Sweden, 1973 to 2009: incidence and risk factors. *J Urol*, 2014, Mar, 191(3), 783-789.

[2] Elliott, CS; Halpern, MS; Paik, J; Maldonado, Y; Shortliffe, LD. Epidemiologic trends in penile anomalies and hypospadias in the state of California, 1985-2006., *J Pediatr Urol*, 2011, Jun, 7(3), 294-298.

[3] Snodgrass, W. Hypospadias. In: Wein A, Kavoussi L, Novick A, Partin A, Peters C, eds. Campbell-Walsh Urology. 10th ed. Philadelphia, PA: *Elsevier Saunders*, 2012, 3503-3536.

[4] Cruz-Diaz, O; Castellan, M; Gosalbez, R. Use of buccal mucosa in hypospadias repair. *Curr Urol Rep*, 2013, Aug, 14(4), 366-372.

[5] Barbagli, G; Vallasciani, S; Romano, G; Fabbri, F; Guazzoni, G; Lazzeri, M. Morbidity of oral mucosa graft harvesting from a single cheek. *Eur Urol*, 2010, Jul, 58(1), 33-41.

[6] Orabi, H; Bouhout, S; Morissette, A; Rousseau, A; Chabaud, S; Bolduc, S. Tissue engineering of urinary bladder and urethra: advances from bench to patients. *Scientific World Journal*, 2013 Dec 24, 2013, 1-13.

[7] Patel, MN; Atala, A. Tissue engineering of the penis. *Scientific World Journal*, 2011, 11, 2567-2578.

[8] Jeong, SI; Kim, BS; Lee, YM; Ihn, KJ; Kim, SH; Kim, YH. Morphology of elastic poly(L-lactide-co-e-caprolactone copolymers and in vitro degradation behavior of their scaffolds. *Biomacromolecules*, 2004, 5(4), 1303-1309.

[9] Jeong, SI; Kim, BS; Kang, SQ; et al.. In vivo biocompatibility and degradation behavior of elastic poly (L-lactide-co-e-caprolactone) scaffolds. *Biomaterials*, 2004, 25(28), 5939-5946.

[10] Hayami, JWS; Surrao, DC; Waldman, SD; Amsden, BG. Design and characterization of a biodegradable composite scaffold for ligament tissue engineering. *Journal of Biomedical Materials Research*, 2010, 92(4), 1407-1420.

[11] Furthmayr, H; Timpl, R. Immunochemistry of collagens and procollagens. *Int Rev Connect Tissue Res*, 1976, 7, 61-99.

[12] Fossum, M; Nordenskjöld, A. Tissue-engineered transplants for the treatment of severe hypospadias. *Horm Res Paediatr*, 2010, 73(2), 148-152.

[13] Chen, F; Yoo, JJ; Atala, A. Acellular collagen matrix as a possible "off the shelf" biomaterial for urethral repair. *Urology*, 1999, Sep, 54(3), 407-410.

[14] Atala, A; Guzman, L; Retik, AB. A novel inert collagen matrix for hypospadias repair. *J Urol*, 1999, Sep, 162(3 Pt 2), 1148-1151.

[15] El-Kassaby, AW; Retik, AB; Yoo, JJ; Atala, A. Urethral stricture repair with an off-the-shelf collagen matrix. *J Urol*, 2003, Jan, 169(1), 170-3.

[16] El-Kassaby, A; AbouShwareb, T; Atala, A. Randomized comparative study between buccal mucosal and acellular bladder matrix grafts in complex anterior urethral strictures. *J Urol*, 2008, Apr, 179(4), 1432-1436.

[17] Donkov, II; Bashir, A; Elenkov, CH; Panchev, PK. Dorsal onlay augmentation urethroplasty with small intestinal submucosa: modified Barbagli technique for strictures of the bulbar urethra. *Int J Urol*, 2006, Nov, 13(11), 1415-1417.

[18] Fiala, R; Vidlar, A; Vrtal, R; Belej, K; Student, V. Porcine small intestinal submucosa graft for repair of anterior urethral strictures. *Eur Urol*, 2007, Jun, 51(6), 1702-8.

[19] Palminteri, E; Berdondini, E; Fusco, F; De Nunzio, C; Salonia, A. Long-term results of small intestinal submucosa graft in bulbar urethral reconstruction. *Urology*, 2012, Mar, 79(3), 695-701.

[20] Dorin, RP; Pohl, HG; De Filippo, RE; Yoo, JJ; Atala, A. Tubularized urethral replacement with unseeded matrices: what is the maximum distance for normal tissue regeneration? World *J Urol*, 2008, Aug, 26(4), 323-326.

[21] Nagele, U; Maurer, S; Feil, G; Bock, C; Krug, J; Sievert, KD; et al. In vitro investigations of tissue-engineered multilayered urothelium

established from bladder washings. *Eur Urol*, 2008, Dec, 54(6), 1414-1422.

[22] Zhang, Y; McNeill, E; Tian, H; Soker, S; Andersson, KE; Yoo, JJ; et al. Urine derived cells are a potential source for urological tissue reconstruction. *J Urol*, 2008, Nov, 180(5), 2226-2233.

[23] Fu, Q; Cao, YL. Tissue engineering and stem cell application of urethroplasty: from bench to bedside. *Urology*, 2012, Feb, 79(2), 246-253.

[24] Gertow, K; Wolbank, S; Rozell, B; Sugars, R; Andang, M; Parish, CL; et al. Organized development from human embryonic stem cells after injection into immunodeficient mice. *Stem Cells Dev*, 2004, Aug, 13(4), 421-435.

[25] Przyborski, SA. Differentiation of human embryonic stem cells after transplantation in immune-deficient mice. *Stem Cells*, 2005, Oct, 23(9), 1242-1250.

[26] Bernardo, ME; Emons, JA; Karperien, M; Nauta, AJ; Willemze, R; Roelofs, H; et al. Human mesenchymal stem cells derived from bone marrow display a better chondrogenic differentiation compared with other sources. *Connect Tissue Res*, 2007, 48(3), 132-140.

[27] Rosland, GV; Svendsen, A; Torsvik, A; Sobala, E; McCormack, E; Immervoll, H; et al. Long-term cultures of bone marrow-derived human mesenchymal stem cells frequently undergo spontaneous malignant transformation. *Cancer Res*, 2009, Jul 1, 69(13), 5331-5339.

[28] Rubio, D; Garcia-Castro, J; Martin, MC; de la Fuente, R; Cigudosa, JC; Lloyd, AC; et al. Spontaneous human adult stem cell transformation. *Cancer Res*, 2005, Apr 15, 65(8), 3035-3039.

[29] Bhargava, S; Patterson, JM; Inman, RD; MacNeil, S; Chapple, CR. Tissue-engineered buccal mucosa urethroplasty-clinical outcomes. *Eur Urol*, 2008 Jun, 53(6), 1263-1269.

[30] De Filippo, RE; Yoo, JJ; Atala, A. Urethral replacement using cell seeded tubularized collagen matrices. *J Urol*, 2002, Oct, 168(4 Pt 2), 1789-1792.

[31] Fu, Q; Deng, CL; Liu, W; Cao, YL. Urethral replacement using epidermal cell-seeded tubular acellular bladder collagen matrix. *BJU Int*, 2007, May, 99(5), 1162-1165.

[32] Orabi, H; AbouShwareb, T; Zhang, Y; Yoo, JJ; Atala, A. Cell-seeded tubularized scaffolds for reconstruction of long urethral defects: a preclinical study. *Eur Urol*, 2013, Mar, 63(3), 531-538.

[33] Raya-Rivera, A; Esquiliano, DR; Yoo, JJ; Lopez-Bayghen, E; Soker, S; Atala, A. Tissue-engineered autologous urethras for patients who need reconstruction: an observational study. *Lancet*, 2011 Apr 2, 377(9772), 1175-1182.

[34] Fossum, M; Svensson, J; Kratz, G; Nordenskjöld, A. Autologous in vitro cultured urothelium in hypospadias repair. *J Pediatr Urol*, 2007, Feb, 3(1), 10-18.

[35] Bouhout, S; Perron, E; Gauvin, R; Bernard, G; Ouellet, G; Cattan, V; et al.. In vitro reconstruction of an autologous, watertight, and resistant vesical equivalent. *Tissue Eng Part A*, 2010, May, 16(5), 1539-1548.

[36] Magnan, M; Levesque, P; Gauvin, R; Dube, J; Barrieras, D; El-Hakim, A; et al.. Tissue engineering of a genitourinary tubular tissue graft resistant to suturing and high internal pressures. *Tissue Eng Part A*, 2009, Jan, 15(1), 197-202.

[37] Rousseau, A; Fradette, J; Bernard, G; Gauvin, R; Laterreur, V; Bolduc, S. Adipose-derived stromal cells for the reconstruction of a human vesical equivalent. *Journal of Tissue Engineering and Regenerative Medicine*, 2013.

[38] Imbeault, A; Bernard, G; Rousseau, A; Morissette, A; Chabaud, S; Bouhout, S; et al. An endothelialized urothelial cell-seeded tubular graft for urethral replacement. *Can Urol Assoc J*, 2013, Jan-Feb, 7(1-2), E4-E9.

In: Hypospadias
Editor: Daniel H. Preston

ISBN: 978-1-63482-023-3

Chapter 4

Urethrocutaneous Fistula after Hypospadias Surgery: To Prevent and to Repair

Mirko Bertozzi*[*], *Niccolò Nardi*, *Marco Prestipino and Antonino Appignani
S. C. di Clinica Chirurgica Pediatrica, Università degli Studi di Perugia, Ospedale S. Maria della Misericordia, Italy

Abstract

Although fistula historically has been the most common complication in hypospadias surgery, with a frequency up to 11%, the incidence has decreased during the last 20 years to less than 5%. Rarely some small fistulas resolve spontaneously. Nonetheless, recurrence is still possible. Many solutions are available to decrease the incidence of fistula, such as use of better suture materials, microsurgical instruments, magnification, silicone catheters or stents, reliable postoperative dressing and vascularized island flaps to protect the neourethra the use of flaps to cover the neourethra has been shown to decrease the incidence. We report

[*] S. C. di Clinica Chirurgica Pediatrica, Università degli Studi di Perugia, Ospedale S. Maria della Misericordia, Loc. S. Andrea delle Fratte, 06100 Perugia, Italy. Tel: + 39-075-5783376. Mob: + 39-339-3196807. Fax: + 39-075-5783376. E-Mail: mirkobertozzi@hotmail.com.

our experience to prevent and to repair urethrocutaneous fistula in hypospadias surgery.

To Prevent

The authors report results of their experience using a personal protection for the neourethra during TIP urethroplasty, a double de-epithelialized preputial flap transposed anteriorly and cross-sutured above the neourethra, or double-cross flap protection. This kind of protection is simple to perform, and the flaps used to protect the urethroplasty are easy to obtain and manipulate. Although the time required to perform our procedure is slightly longer offers an unquestionable advantage in complication rate, especially concerning fistula occurrence.

To Repair

Fistulae appear in areas of least resistance of the reconstructed urethra because of an inadequate cicatrisation process and/or due to infective processes that are often related to an insufficient blood supply. However, most fistulae require a further surgical procedure, where the risk of recurrence is almost the same. The authors describe the urethrocutaneous fistula repair after urethroplasty using *n*-butyl-cyanoacrylate (*N*BCA) in an outpatient setting. In this experience the use of *N*BCA as a minimally invasive treatment for fistula repair gave good results for repairing fistulae with a success rate of 50%. The results encourage the use of *N*BCA as a first non-surgical attempt to repair urethrocutaneous fistulae especially if the fistula is 2 mm. The failure of this procedure does not compromise a possible subsequent surgical repair.

Surgical repair performed by authors is a re-TIP urethroplasty with a double de-epithelialized preputial flap as described for the primary repair. This kind of procedure for hypospadias reoperation in a previously circumcised patient with a failed hypospadias does not show a significant difference from the techniques described for primary repair.

Vascular reinforcement flaps supply additional blood flow, supporting the wound's healing, and avoids fistula in poor vascularity areas, such as in secondary cases.

Introduction

Urethrocutaneous fistula represents one of the most frequent causes of morbidity in urethroplasty. Hypospadias can be repaired using different surgical techniques but, regardless of the technique, incidences of recurrent fistula are reported with a rate of 10-15% associated with one-stage repairs [1]. The frequency of fistula has decreased in the last two decades and its incidence may be used to judge the success of the operation for hypospadias' defect [2]; a 5% fistula rate is usually anticipated [3]. The surgical repair of a fistula remains the treatment of choice, even if some patients need further operations because of recurrences. Ritcher et al. [4] in their experience reported a range of fistula re-operation of 2-15%.

The aetiology of fistula and wound dehiscence has been a controversial issue in paediatric urology. Several factors, such as suture material, infection, previous operations, catheterization and surgical skill may significantly affect outcomes. Various procedures have been developed to avoid the occurrence of fistula formation. Various procedures have been developed to avoid the occurrence of fistula formation and many strategies have been taken to repair the same if appeared in the post operative period. Here we report our experience in preventing fistula formation after hypospadias surgery and in repair it if occurred.

Fistula Formation after Hypospadias Surgery

To Prevent

Since it was first described by Snodgrass [5] in 1994, tubularized incised plate (TIP) urethroplasty had a worldwide diffusion. However, urethrocutaneous fistula is still reported as the most frequent complication [6, 7].

One of the most important factors to avoid the occurrence of fistula is the application of a protective intermediate layer of tissue between the neourethra and the skin [8]. In fact, flapless urethroplasties have a higher risk of fistula development [9]. Using TIP urethroplasty in conjunction with a protective layer of tissue to cover the suture line can help to prevent fistula formation, either in first correction of hypospadias or in reoperative urethroplasty [8, 10,

11]. Smith in 1973 described first de-epithelialized flap [12]. The principle was later applied by Belman [13] demonstrating that the layer between the neourethra and skin provides a remarkable contribution to hypospadias repair.

The use of a protective intermediate layer as external spermatic fascia flap, tunica vaginalis, scrotal and ventral dartos flaps have been described as alternatives to the dorsal ones especially in circumcised boys or those undergoing reoperation [8, 14-16].

Finally the use of adjacent spongiosum tissue to reinforce the neourethra as second-layer coverage [17] is reported but it is limited especially in mid-shaft and proximal hypospadias.

Some authors have reported no incidence of fistula after hypospadias repair with single overlay [10, 18]. Others using only single flap for urethral coverage report an incidence of fistula ranging from 4.8% to 14%. [19, 20]. However, urethrocutaneous fistulas represent the most frequent complication [6, 7] and the reported incidence is as high as 2-16% [21-22].

It is not clear how urethrocutaneous fistula develops in presence of an interposed flap. Moreover, when a SDF is used, a fistula track can develop through the suture line next to the flap edge. Fistula can find the way through a small perforation of flap due to injury during dissection, focal ischemic injury or infection.

The first author to publish a double dartos flap (DDF) to protect the neourethra was Kamal in 2005 [23], affirming that DDF provides more protection against fistula development rather than a single flap. This seals the neourethra from the glans and skin on the front, as well as on both sides, and provides more protection against fistulas development. When DDF are fashioned, a possible damage of the first flap which may cause fistulas, would be protected by the second one.

Since this date, other authors have reported their experience in covering the neourethra with a double layer of dartos tissue in TIP urethroplasty, with very similar techniques and excellent results [24-28]. In 2011 a multicentric experience about this topic was published [29].

The Double-cross Flap Protection Technique [26]

In this technique after creating the neourethra via TIP urethroplasty (Figures 1-3) the de-epithelialized preputial flap is prepared as a transverse island flap. Transillumination is used to pinpoint the course of the vascular supply. Using straight scissors, a longitudinal incision is made along the vascularized flap to create 2 halves (Figure 4).

The 2 halves are deepithelialized, the cutis is removed and the vascular pedicles are preserved. The halves are then ventrally rotated over the neourethra, 1 to the right and 1 to the left. Continuous or interrupted sutures can then be used to fix the flaps to the neourethra. The first flap is positioned longitudinally over the neourethra as far as 1 cm beneath the native hypospadic meatus and sutured along both sides of the neourethra with 2 continuous polyglactin 7-zero sutures (Figure 5).

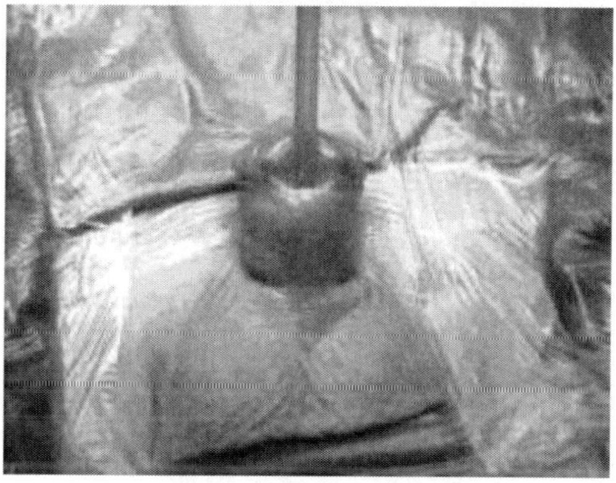

Figure 1. Distal hypospadias.

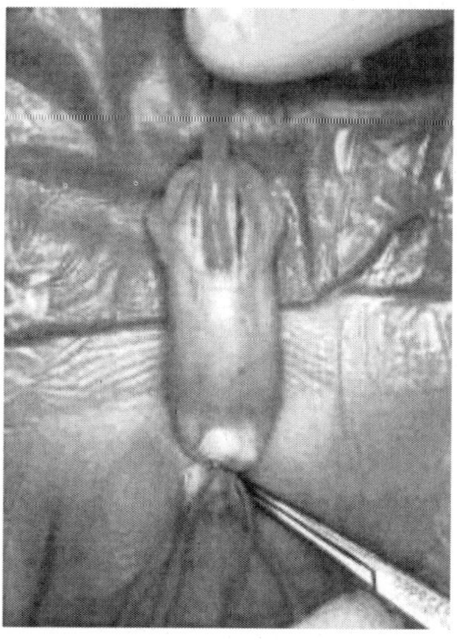

Figure 2. The peri meatal and peri urethral plate tissue are incised.

The second flap is transposed transversely exactly over the first flap, covering it entirely (Figure 6).

Interrupted sutures of the same material are used. This approach creates a double-cross flap on the neourethra but the sutures of the 2 flaps do not overlap each other (Figure 7).

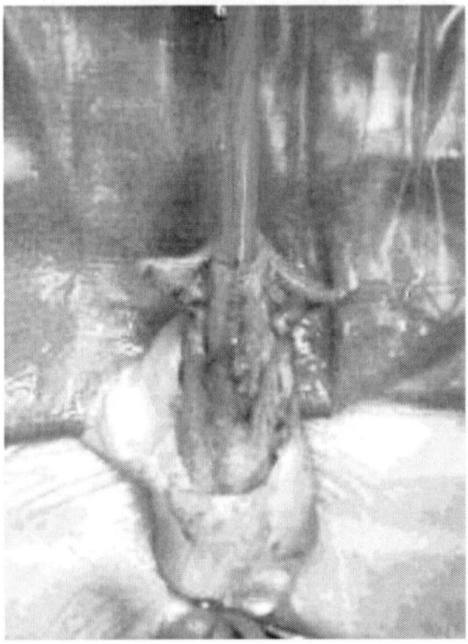

Figure 3. TIP urethroplasty.

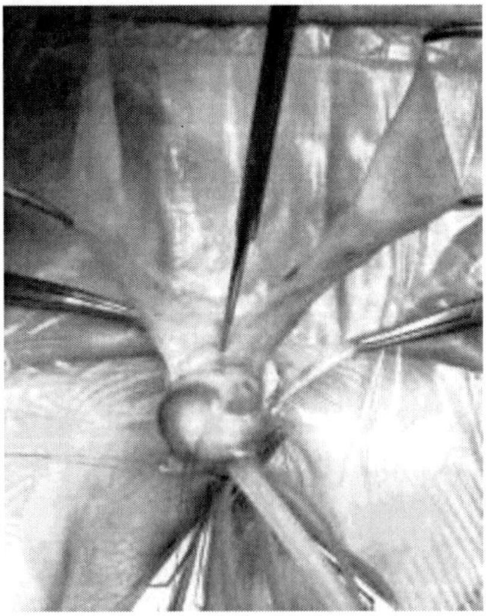

Figure 4. Longitudinal incision is made along flap to create 2 hemi-flaps.

The glans and skin are closed conventionally. Surgical time is 90 to 120 minutes. In all cases we used 6-zero and 7-zero polyglactin sutures well lubricated with petroleum jelly and microsurgical instruments with a 2.5X optical magnification. The urethroplasty was prepared using a Foley catheter (6Ch or 8Ch for younger patients, 10Ch for older patients) and a compressive dressing was applied. Patients were discharged home the following day. On postoperative day 4 the dressing was removed and a noncompressive dressing was applied. On postoperative day 7 the urethral catheter and dressing were removed at the outpatient department.

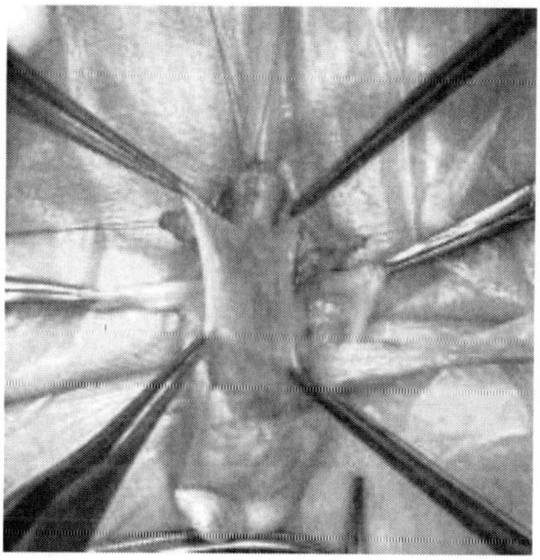

Figure 5. First flap is placed longitudinally to cover neourethra in its entirety.

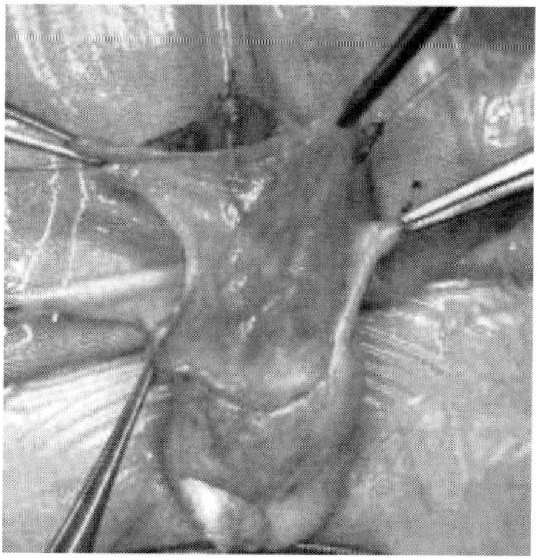

Figure 6. Second flap is transversely superimposed over first flap.

Personal Experience

A total of 103 children 12 months to 10 years old (mean 39 months) underwent TIP urethroplasty with DCFP between October 2005 and September 2012. All patients were submitted to the intervention for distal and mid shaft hypospadias.

Ventral curvature was present in 19 patients. No patient had previously undergone urethroplasty.

We evaluated retrospectively analyzing results the double-cross flap protection technique.

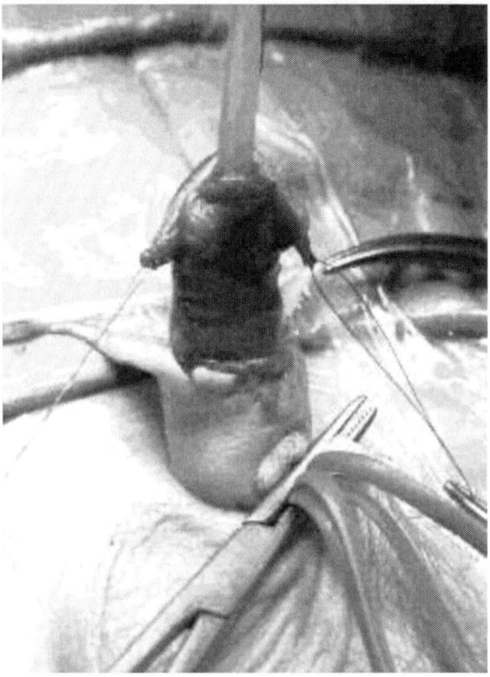

Figure 7. Double-cross flap is created on neourethra. Sutures do not overlap each other.

Results

19 children presented ventral curvature, which resolved in 4 following the Nesbit procedure and in 15 following excision of the ventral chordee.

3 patient exhibited fistula at follow up (2.5%). Of these fistulae, one resolved spontaneously, another one was repaired by application of cyanoacrlate [30, 31] and the last needed a new intervention. In 2 patients a glandular dehiscence of the urethroplasty occurred (1.7%).

Mild stenosis of the neomeatus occurred in 3 patients (2.5%), which was treated and resolved with dilations at home for 15 to 20 days using a self-lubricating catheter of the same caliber as the urinary catheter used for urethroplasty.

The catheter was inserted just above the native hypospadic meatus for 15 minutes twice daily. All dilations were performed by parents of the patients, who had received training. Follow up was 20 to 34 months and no recurrence was observed.

In our experience comparing these results of double-cross flap protection technique with patients previously treated with TIP urethroplasty with no protection and TIP urethroplasty with the Retik approach the incidence of fistulas decreased from 15% using TIP urethroplasty with no protection to 10% using TIP urethroplasty with the Retik approach and to 2.5% with our technique. Nevertheless considering that one in one patient the fistula recovered spontaneously the percentage of fistula decrease to 1.7%.

Comment

It is well known that fistulae appear in areas of least resistance of the reconstructed urethra because of an inadequate cicatrization process and/or due to infective processes that are often related to a poor blood supply.

In the double-cross flap protection technique to preserve as much blood supply as possible to the flap, its dissection from the shaft skin did not go beyond 1 to 2 cm distal to the root of the penis.

We think that the double well vascularized flap interposed between the neourethra and the skin might have a very good blood supply for the neourethra. Meatal stenosis is another complication that may be observed after TIP procedure.

Literature indicates the occurrence of metal stenosis is between 0.7 and 17% after TIP repair [32, 33]. Lorenzo and Snodgrass reported that the dorsal midline incision wound was healed without cicatricial evidence and did not cause meatal and urethral stenosis [32]. However, tight closing of the distal neourethra could cause a narrow meatus [33].

In our experience we had only 3 mild stenosis (2.5%). In all cases stenoses are limited to the meatus and they were managed by simple meatal dilation and none of these cases required meatotomy.

Dehiscence in presence of the dartos flap is a rare complication but Elbakry [9] claimed that the dartos flap should not be used because it hinders tension-free closure of the glans flaps and increases the risk of glanular dehiscence. We believe that the drawback of the double-cross flap protection technique might be the great thickness of tissue that may make approximation and closure of the glanular wings difficult. Therefore the presence of a the double-cross flap protection to protect the neourethra could have a greater risk of glanular dehiscence.

In the present case series glanular dehiscence was seen only in 2 cases (1.7) probably due to the limited experience of some surgeons. To avoid this complication we claim that glans wings must be widely separated and generously deepened to obtaining good mobility for later closure. Nevertheless dehiscence limited to the glans occurred in two cases of repaired midpenile hypospadias which need re-intervention.

Penile rotation may be another possible complication after TIP urethroplasty using a single flap carried out with a transverse island of dorsal subcutaneous tissue to protect the neourethra as described by Retik. Limiting factors as poor developed ventral skins, insufficient flap length and asymmetric flap were reported to be cause of penile rotation.

Snodgrass originally describes its technique protected by a transverse island of dorsal subcutaneous tissue used as a flap [5], Later on, probably for the possibility of penile rotation Snodgrass transposed the flap ventrally in a buttonhole fashion to cover the neourethra [34].

In a well fashioned TIP urethroplasty protected by the double-cross flap protection both flaps are ventrally rotated and transposed over the neourethra, with symmetric rotation and equal tension trying to avoid penile rotation.

In this experience penile rotation did not occur.

The eventual limitation in performing the double-cross flap protection technique is level of confidence with island flaps. However, the double-cross flap protection technique might be an alternative technique to decrease the fistula rate. Our results are encouraging, and confirm the safety and validity of our procedure.

The double-cross flap protection technique is simple to perform, and the flaps used to protect the urethroplasty are easy to obtain and manipulate. Although the time required to perform our procedure is slightly longer than that required to protect the urethra with a single flap, the double-cross flap protection technique offers an unquestionable advantage in terms of reducing the rate of postoperative fistulas. Based on our results, TIP urethroplasty with the double-cross flap protection has become our procedure of choice for all cases of subcoronal, distal penile shaft and mid shaft hypospadias.

Fistula Formation after Hypospadias Surgery

To Repair

The goal of hypospadias surgery is to restore the urethral meatus to its normal position on the glans, to correct penile curvature and to create a urethra which allows micturition with a controlled stream. According to many authors, children submitted to urethroplasty who do not develop a fistula during follow-up may be considered a success [1].

Many authors report that the incidence of fistula changes depending on the urethroplasty technique used, varying from 0.5% to 10% for the meatal advancement and glanuloplasty technique [35], from 2.2% to 35% for the 'flip-flap' techniques [36, from 1% to 16.7% for the urethral advancement in distal hypospadias [37, 38], from 4% to 33% for the island pedicle tubed repairs [39] and from 15% to 35% for free graft-tubed repairs [40]. Using a two-stage repair Smith [41] reduced his incidence of fistula to < 3% and Greenfield et al. [42] reported a fistula rate of 2.5% using a two-stage modified Belt-Fuqua repair for severe hypospadias with chordee.

Fistulae appear in areas of least resistance of the reconstructed urethra because of an inadequate cicatrisation process and/or due to infective processes that are often related to an insufficient blood supply. Occasionally fistulae occur proximal to a stenotic segment of the neourethra. Fistulae are classified according to size, small (< 2 mm) or large (> 2 mm) [43], and they can recover spontaneously during the first few months after a hypospadias surgical procedure [44]. However, most fistulae require a further surgical procedure, where the risk of recurrence is almost the same. It was reported that treatment with dihydrotestosterone transdermal gel before urethroplasty may reduce the incidence of fistula [45]. Broad spectrum antibiotic prophylaxis appears to be effective in reducing the rate of fistula and stenosis in TIP [46]. Ulman et al. [47] reported that the use of a continuous suture of subcuticular tissue with polydioxanone reduces the incidence of fistula. The fistula repair can be carried out 6-12 months after urethroplasty if its size is < 2 mm using a multilayer simple closure technique. Rotational and advancement skin flaps with suprapubic diversion or three-fold suture with a subcuticular flap may be used to protect the closure for fistula of > 2 mm or multiple ones [48, 49].

Despite all these devices and the different possible techniques for the repair of fistula, the risk of recurrence represents a further challenge for surgeons. Shankar et al. [50] recommended that tissues from an unscarred area (tunica vaginalis or scrotal dartos layer) should be used to cover the repaired fistula to prevent recurrence. Fibrin glue was used as the sealant in hypospadias surgery but did not eliminate fistula formation, although it does minimize its incidence.

Outpatient Department Repair of Urethrocutaneous Fistulae Using *N*-Butyl-Cyanoacrylate (*N*BCA) [30]

Cyanoacrylates are tissue glues that polymerize upon contact with blood or water, creating a tight closure. Their use, in the form of octyl or butyl-cyanoacrylate, has widely increased in the past 10 years [51] in paediatrics for closure of tension-free wounds and has been frequently used as an alternative to conventional sutures. Usages include the management of low fistula-inano [52], treatment of ano-rectal fistula [53], endoscopic treatment in the first episode of varicocele bleeding [54], sutureless circumcision [55] and the closure of laparoscopic trocar-site wounds [56].

The first authors describing fistulae repair with cyanoacrylates were Lapointe et al. [57] in 'early' fistulae. Here we report our experience using *n*-butyl-cyanoacrylate (*N*BCA) glue to repair 'early' and long-standing fistulae after urethroplasty.

Application of N*BCA: Technique*

Early fistulae: Fistula developed within 2-3 days after catheter removal A direct application of *N*BCA, with no sedation or anaesthesia, was performed after the fistulae were disinfected with 10% iodopovidone solution. The application of multilayered *N*BCA was performed directly over the fistulae, carefully approximating the borders of the fistula. During the application a tubular silicone stent was kept in the urethra and removed 10 min after the procedure.

Long-standing fistulae: Fistula that occurred 6-24 months after the initial intervention. A topical anaesthetic (lidocaine 2.5% + prilocaine 2.5% cream) was applied over the fistula after its disinfection with a 10% iodopovidone solution. Then 45 min later all the edges of the fistula was scarified with a 27 G 1.3 cm needle. A multilayer of *N*BCA was then applied, attaching the edges of the fistula. A tubular silicone stent was kept *in situ* just for the application of *N*BCA. The entire procedure took 15 min.

Personal Experience

From January 2003 to December 2012, 16 patients (mean age 36 months) were treated at our outpatients' department for urethrocutaneous fistula which occurred after hypospadias repair. We analyzed the data dividing the patients in two groups: Group A, eight children (mean age 22.6 months) that developed a fistula within two days from the catheter removal following urethroplasty ("early" fistula); Group B, eight children (mean age 42.6 months), who came to our attention presenting with long standing fistula. In all patients, a multilayer of *n*-butyl-cyanoacrilate was applied, attaching the edges of the fistula taking care to perform a scarification of the fistula's edges in patients of Group B before the application of the glue.

In *Group A* three children were affected by subcoronal hypospadias and five presented with an anterior shaft; in all children, fistula occurred on the same site of the native hypospadic meatus. The fistulae were < 2 mm in six cases (one subcoronal and five anterior shaft) and > 2 mm in the remaining subcoronal cases.

Group B comprised seven children who had previously undergone urethroplasty in different surgical centres (mean age 42.6 months) [range 21-84] and came to our attention presenting with long-standing fistulae that occurred 6-24 months after the initial intervention. All the children had undergone TIP urethroplasty (one midshaft and seven subcoronals). The fistulae were < 2 mm in two cases (one midshaft and one subcoronal) and were > 2 mm in the remaining six cases and, as for group A the fistula occurred on the same site of the native meatus.

Table 1. Details of fistulae sites and results of NCBA application(s) in groups A ('early' fistula)

Patient no.	Fistula size, mm	Site of fistula	Applications *N*BCA, *n*	Result
1	≤2MM	Subcoronal	1	Resolution
2	≤2MM	Anterior shaft	3	Failed
3	≤2MM	Anterior Shaft	2	Resolution
4	>2MM	Subcoronal	1	Resolution
5	≤2MM	Anterior Shaft	5	Failed
6	≤2MM	Anterior Shaft	1	Resolution
7	≤2MM	Anterior Shaft	2	Resolution
8	>2MM	Subcoronal	3	Failed

Table 2. Details of fistulae sites and results of NCBA application(s) in groups B (long-standing fistula)

Patient no.	Fistula size, mm	Site of fistula	Applications *N*BCA, *n*	Result
1	≤ 2mm	Subcoronal	3	Resolution
2	> 2mm	Subcoronal	7	Failed
3	> 2mm	Subcoronal	5	Failed
4	≤ 2mm	Anterior shaft	3	Resolution
5	> 2mm	Subcoronal	4	Failed
6	> 2mm	Subcoronal	3	Resolution
7	> 2mm	Subcoronal	5	Failed
8	> 2mm	Subcoronal	3	Failed

Results

In Group A the number of applications *N*BCA was one in three patients and varied from two to a maximum of five in the remaining five.

In Group B the number of applications was always three or more.

Considering all 16 children that underwent the procedure (Group A+B), eight patients had fistula resolution with application of *N*BCA; consisting of five patients in group A (follow-up 5-7 years) and three in group B (follow-up ranges from 1.5-5 years).

In the remaining six patients applications of *N*BCA were ineffective in repairing the fistula (three patients in group A and five in group B) and thus they underwent surgical repair.

The size and site of fistulae, number of applications of NCBA and results of treatment are shown in Tables 1 & 2.

Comment

Cyanoacrylates are monomers that polymerize quickly when hydrogen ions are present, creating an acrylic resin, which solidifies in about 1 min. They exist in two forms: Short-chain cyanoacrylates (methyl-2 or ethyl-2) that are rarely used, because they degrade quickly in to cyanoacrylate and formaldehyde that is very toxic for tissues [58]; and the long-chain cyanoacrylates (*n*-butyl-2-cyanoacrylate and *n*-octyl-2-cyanoacrylate) that degrade slowly, thus build-up of toxic products is minimal, resulting in their being safe for topical skin closure [59]. Cyanoacrylates have become widely used globally since the 2004 Cochrane Database Report [30], which stated that surgeons should consider tissue glue as an alternative to traditional suturing material as it is as effective for infection or leakage. *Ex vivo* studies have not shown any tensiometer difference between classical suture materials and cyanoacrylates [60]. In the present study the glue stay-time varied from a minimum of 4 to a maximum of 7 days, without any differences between group A and B. The edges of the fistula held tight together due to the tensile strength of the cyanoacrylate. These edges are different in relation to the kind of fistula with the 'early' fistulae having granulation tissue, while the long-standing fistula edges are cicatrized.

Scarification of long-standing fistulae edges (group B) produces bleeding tissue, which initiates a new granulation process. The tensile strength of cyanoacrylate maintains the contact of the edges of the fistula favouring the healing process. Moreover *N*BCA provides a waterproof barrier from the underlying urine supporting the granulating process of the edges of the fistula. In the present study, the fistula healed in eight of 16 children (Group A + B) (50%) treated by application of *N*BCA. In the remaining eight failed cases the glue therapy did not compromise the subsequent successful surgical repair [61].

The present experience shows that with this procedure fistula of < 2 mm were more easily repaired than fistulae of > 2 mm. Our method of treatment was more effective in treating the fistulae in group A than Group B. It seems that the fistula site is irrelevant for the success of this therapy. Moreover from this preliminary study it appears that fistulae which tend to recover are those that respond to the very first applications.

Although we obtained good results with the application of *N*BCA to repair fistula after urethroplasty, obviously the best result is to reduce the incidence of fistula development after hypospadias surgery. A good quality surgery at the time of the initial operation and the interposition of tissue between the epithelium of the neourethra and the epithelium of the skin can reduce the incidence of this complication [13, 26-29].

In conclusion, the gold standard for the treatment of urethrocutaneous fistula is surgical repair. *N*BCA provides rapid healing with a good watertight closure. It is feasible with or without topical anaesthesia in the outpatients setting and it is repeatable. In our experience this treatment reduces parents' anxiety because it represents the possibility for early resolution without any surgical procedure under general anaesthesia. From our obtained results we encourage the use of *N*BCA as a first non-surgical attempt to repair 'early' and long-standing urethrocutaneous fistulae especially if the fistula is < 2 mm because the failure of this procedure does not compromise a possible subsequent surgical repair.

Double-cross Flap Protection Technique for Fistula and Dehiscence Repair [61]

Reoperation for failed hypospadias has been considered to be seriously problematic. The dense fibrotic tissue causes difficulties in wound healing and increases the rate of complications. The TIP urethroplasty method has become a preferred method for all varieties of hypospadias in the past decade. However, fistulas are still one of the most common complications of this technique. Results of this procedure were already published in a recent publication [61].

Technique

For previously circumcised patients, lateral penile skin flaps were mobilized for the harvesting of dartos tissue and penile shaft skin coverage. In patients suffering from a breakdown of a previous hypospadias repair, any skin irregularity was corrected for better evaluation of the presenting defect and proper performance of the re-operative repair. After a traction suture was placed through the glans, a skin incision was carried out around the urethral plate, and a perimeatal incision was also made on the ventrum. Two parallel incisions were made to define the urethral plate, and the glans wings were elevated.

The urethral plate was incised along the midline, including the mucosal and submucosal tissue from within the meatus to the tip of the urethral plate, and the plate was tubularised with 7/0 absorbable full thickness running suture. After a sufficient de-gloving of the penis and tubularisation of the plate, traction sutures were placed on the borders of the inner face of the ventral-side skin. The de-epithelialised dartos flaps were bilaterally prepared from the adjacent residual dartos fascia and completely de-epithelialised, with the dissection of the outer surface of the penile skin. Vascularised ventral dartos flaps harvested from each side of the penis were brought with their vascular supply. They were transposed to cover the suture line by wrapping them from either side of the penis. Both of the flaps were sutured to the ventral side of the penile shaft and inner glanular wing conjunctions on each counter side (Figures 8-9-10).

Finally, the glanular wings were symmetrically closed over the overlapping dartos flaps with 7-0 polydioxanone sutures in two layers. A foley catheter (6-10F), corresponding to the diameter of the native urethra, was left in place for seven days for all patients (Figure 11).

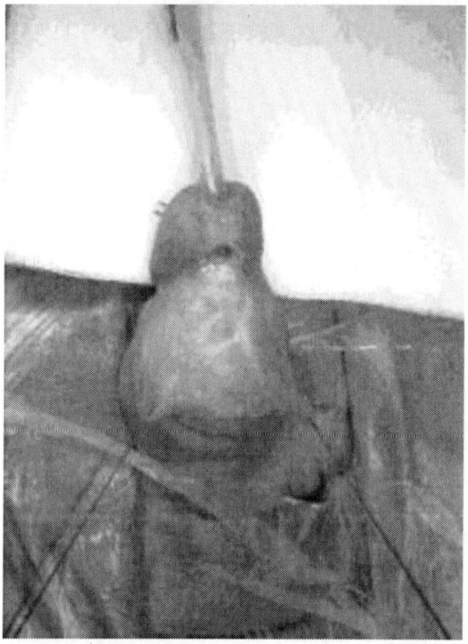

Figure 8. Presence of fistula > 3mm.

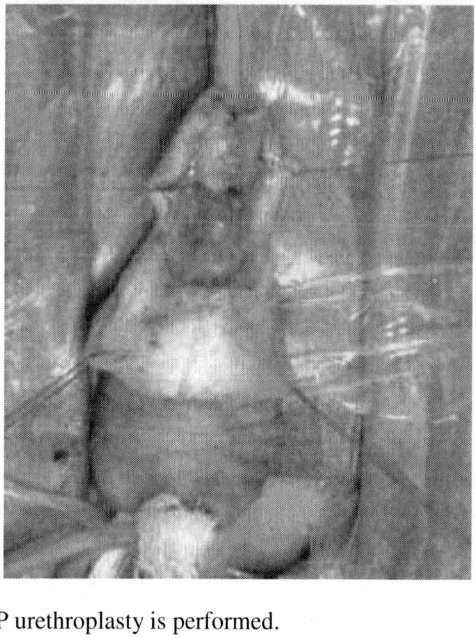

Figure 9. A new TIP urethroplasty is performed.

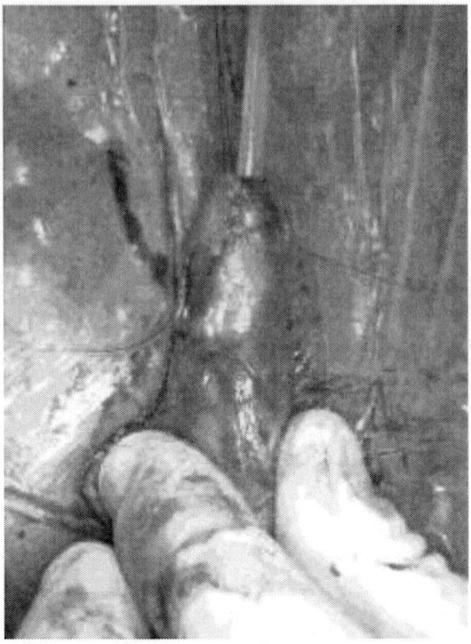

Figure 10. Appearance of the two flaps applied.

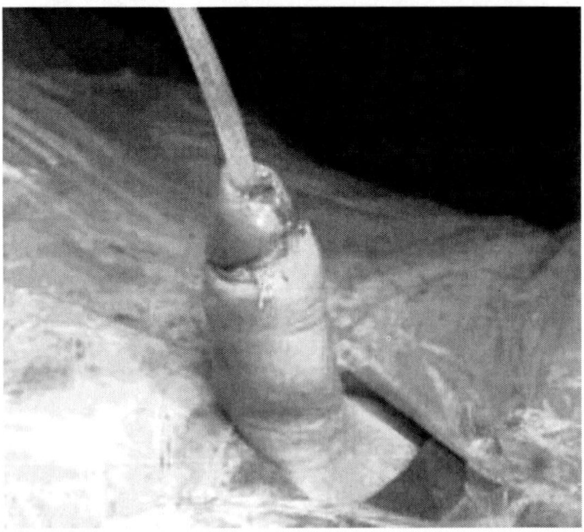

Figure 11. Immediate post-operative aspect of the penis.

Personal Experience

Between February 2009 and August 2014, a total of 12 patients were subjected to TIP urethroplasty with double de-epithelised dartos flaps for the correction of complications related to previous hypospadias surgery.

The mean follow-up time was 26 months (range of 12-65 months). The mean age of the patients was 3.9 (range of 2 to 8 years). At the time of repair, the location of the meatus was observed as coronal in 8 patients, sub-coronal in 2 patients, and mid-penile in two patients. All patients had been previously circumcised. No chordee was observed in any case. Ten cases were admitted to our institutions with complaint of wound dehiscence all along the suture lines and two cases with major fistula (more than 3 mm).

All patients having an initial TIP urethroplasty were re-operated, using TIP urethroplasty with double-cross flap protection.

Two of the cases were operated with the TIP urethroplasty procedure twice before being admitted to our institution.

Results

All patients who underwent a secondary TIP urethroplasty with double-cross flap protection procedures were successfully repaired. Devascularisation of the overlaying skin from which dartos separated was not observed. No postoperative complications occurred except in one case (new dehiscence). We achieved satisfactory results in all secondary cases by using TIP urethroplasty with double-cross flap protection.

Comment

Complications are common after hypospadias repair, ranging from minor fistulas to complete loss of the neourethra, requiring total reconstruction. The fistula incidence rate in secondary operations in failed hypospadias repairs have been reported as higher than in primary cases. [62]

Although Telfer et al. and Borer et al. reported that using a protective intermediate layer reduced the fistula rate from 63% to 4.5%, [63] some researchers reported high fistula rates despite the use of a single dartos flap as a barrier layer. [6, 14, 64] Recently, in a study done by Yigiter et al., the authors compared the complication rates of the flapless, single flap, double flaps and procedures in TIP urethroplasty, and reported a 29.4%, 26% and 0.1% incidence of fistulas, respectively. [65] In our previous studies, we concluded that TIPU with double dartos flaps seems far more effective in completely covering the neourethra than the methods including a single flap. [26]

The reason for fistula development is not well known in single dartos flaps covering the neourethra. The fistula tract can find its way through a small perforation due to injury during dissection, a focal ischemic injury, infection of the edges of the flap. When double dartos flaps are used, a perforation in one flap that may cause an urethrocutaneous fistula would be protected by the second-layer dartos flap.

TIP urethroplasty with double de-epithelised dartos flaps for hypospadias reoperation in a previously circumcised patient with a failed hypospadias does not show a significant difference from the techniques described for primary repair.

The blood to the urethral plate is supplied by both urethral and deep dorsal arteries. Although the urethral plate is incised in the midline as part of the Snodgrass technique, this does not interrupt or significantly alter the dual blood supply to the two newly-mobile and easily-tubularised strips. For these reasons, TIP urethroplasty seems to be the most suitable re-operative method for cases with failed hypospadias.

If a preputial dartos flap is not available, as in all of our cases where the patient had been previously circumcised, an approximation of adjacent tissues alongside the neourethra can be used as an adequate substitute in a double dartos flaps fashion.

We found the harvesting of the flaps easier, due to the release of the chordee in the previous operations. It was not necessary to de-glove the penis completely as in primary cases. Limited dissection of the dartos flaps from the adjacent tissues was found adequate to cover the whole suture line. This limited dissection can also preserve the circulation of the ventral penile skin. As we know, disrupted vascular circulation in secondary cases can increase wound-healing time and complication rates. Additional blood flow and a nutritious layer of neourethra due to vascular reinforcement flaps were estimated to be extremely important factors in a condition with limited blood flow, such as re-operation areas. The low rates of complications in our reoperation hypospadias cases can be related to the fact that the dartos flap is strong enough and has abundant vascular structure.

It can be estimated that the risk of glandular wound dehiscence is suspected to be higher in patients who have double dartos flaps than in those patients who have only one-layer covering. [65] Glans closure was comfortably achieved and wound dehiscence was seen only in one case. In conclusion, we think that TIP urethroplasty with double-cross flap protection is very efficacious in preventing fistula formation, even in reoperation in failed hypospadias cases. Vascular reinforcement flaps supply additional blood flow, supporting the wound's healing, and avoids fistulas and dehiscence in poor vascularization areas, such as in secondary cases.

References

[1] Baskin L. S. Hypospadias. In Grosfeld J. L., O'Neill J. A. Jr., Fonkalsrud E. W., Coran A. G. eds, *Pediatric Surgery,* Vol. 2. Philadelphia: Mosby Elsevier, 2006: 1870-98.

[2] Retik A. B., Keating M., Mandell J. Complications of hypospadias repair. *Urol Clin North Am* 1988; 15: 223-36.

[3] Belman A. B. Editorial comment. *J Urol* 1994; 152: 1237.

[4] Richter F., Pinto P. A., Stock J. A., Hanna M. K. Management of recurrent urethral fistulas after hypospadias repair. *Urology* 2003; 61: 448-51.

[5] Snodgrass W. Tubularized, incised plate urethroplasty for distal hypospadias. *J Urol* 1994151:464-465.

[6] Sozubir S., Snodgrass W. A new algorithm for primary hypospadias repair based on tip urethroplasty. *J Pediatr Surg* 2003 38:1157-61.

[7] Snodgrass W. T. Snodgrass technique for hypospadias repair. *BJU Int* 2005; 95:683-93.

[8] Hayashi Y., Kojima Y., Kurokawa S. et al., Scrotal dartos flap for the prevention of the urethrocutaneous fistula on hypospadias urethroplasty. *Int J Urol* 2005; 12: 280-3.

[9] Elbakry A. Tubularized-incised urethral plate urethroplasty: Is regular dilatation neccessary for success? *BJU Int* 1999 84: 683-8.

[10] Djordjevic M. L., Perovic S. V., Slavkovic Z. et al., Longitudinal dorsal dartos flap for prevention of fistula after a Snodgrass hypospadias procedure. *Eur Urol* 2006; 50: 53-7.

[11] Baccala A. A. Jr., Ross J., Detore N. et al., Modified tubularized incised plate urethroplasty (Snodgrass) procedure for hypospadias repair. *Urology* 2005; 66:1305-6.

[12] Smith E. D. A de-epithelialized overlap flap technique in the repair of hypospadias. *Br J Plast Surg* 1973; 26: 106-114.

[13] Belman A. B. The de-epithelialized flap and its influence on hypospadias repair. *J Urol* 1994; 152: 2332-4.

[14] Chatterjee U. S., Mandal M. K., Basu S. et al., Comparative study of dartos fascia and tunica vaginalis pedicle wrap for the tubularized incised plate in primary hypospadias repair. *BJU Int* 2004; 94:1102-4.

[15] Soygur T., Arikan N., Zumrutbas A. E. et al., Snodgrass hypospadias repair with ventral based dartos flap in combination with mucosal collars. *Eur Urol* 2005; 47: 879-84.

[16] Yamataka A., Ando K., Lane G. J. et al., Pedicled external spermatic fascia flap for urethroplasty in hypospadias and closure of urethrocutaneous fistula. *J Pediatr Surg* 1998 33:1788-9.
[17] Snodgrass W., Koyle M., Manzoni G. et al., Tubularized incised plate hypospadias repair for proximal hypospadias. *J Urol* 1998; 159: 2129-31.
[18] Retik A. B., Mandell J., Bauer S. B. et al., Meatal based hypospadias repair with the use of a dorsal subcutaneous flap to prevent urethrocutaneous fistula. *J Urol* 1994; 152: 1229-31.
[19] Al Hunayan A. A., Kehinde E. O., Elsalam M. A. et al., Tubularized incised plate urethroplasty: Modification and outcome. *Int Urol Nephrol* 2003; 35: 47-52.
[20] Tonvichien L. and Niramis R. Tubularized, incised plate urethroplasty in hypospadias repair: Experience at Queen Sirikit National Institute of Child Health. *J Med Assoc Thai* 2003; 86: S522-30.
[21] Sugarman I. D., Trevett J., Malone P. S. Tubularization of the incised urethral plate (Snodgrass procedure) for primary hypospadias surgery. *BJU Int* 1999; 83:88-90.
[22] Guralnick M. L., al-Shammari A., Williot P. E. et al., Outcome of hypospadias repair using the tubularized, incised plate urethroplasty. *Can J Urol* 2000; 7:986-991.
[23] Kamal B. A., Double dartos flaps in tubularized incised plate hypospadias repair. *Urology* 2005; 66:1095-1098.
[24] Bakan V., Yildiz A. Dorsal double-layer dartos flap for preventing fistulae formation in the Snodgrass technique. *Urol Int* 2007; 78:241-244.
[25] Mustafa M., Wadie B. S., Abol-Enein H., Standard Snodgrass technique in conjunction with double-layer covering of the neourethra with dorsal dartos flap is the therapy of first choice for hypospadias. *Int Urol Nephrol* 2008; 40:573-576.
[26] Appignani A., Prestipino M., Bertozzi M. et al., Double-cross flap protection: new technique for coverage of neourethra in hypospadias repair. *J Urol* 2009; 182:1521-1527.
[27] Erol A., Kayikci A., Memik O. et al., Single vs double dartos interposition flaps in preventing urethrocutaneous fistula after tubularized incised plate urethroplasty in primary distal hypospadias: A prospective randomized study. *Urol Int* 2009; 83:354-358.

[28] Abolyosr A., Snodgrass hypospadias repair with onlay overlapping double layered dorsal dartos flap without urethrocutaneous fistula: Experience of 156 cases. *J Pediatr Urol* 2010; 6:403-407.

[29] Bertozzi M., Yıldız A., Kamal B., Mustafa M., Prestipino M., Yiğiter M., Al-Darawany H., Oral A., Nardi N., Appignani A. Multicentric experience on double dartos flap protection in tubularized incised plate urethroplasty for distal and midpenile hypospadias. *Pediatr Surg Int.* 2011;27:1331-6.

[30] Prestipino M., Bertozzi M., Nardi N., Appignani A., Outpatient department repair of urethrocutaneous fistulae using *n*-butyl-cyanoacrylate (*N*BCA): A single-centre experience. *BJU Int.* 2011; 108:1514-7.

[31] Bertozzi M., Appignani A., Applications of cyanoacrylate glue in pediatric urology. *N Am J Med Sci.* 2012; 4:323-4.

[32] Lorenzo A. J., Snodgrass W. T. Regular dilatation is unnecessary after tabularized incised-plate hypospadias repair. *BJU Int* 2002; 89:94-7.

[33] Stehr M., Lehner M., Schuster T. et al., Tubularized incised plate (TIP) urethroplasty (Snodgrass) in primary hypospadias repair. *Eur J Pediatr Surg* 2005; 15:420-4.

[34] Snodgrass W. T. Tubularized incised plate (TIP) hypospadias repair. *Urol Clin North Am* 2002; 29:285-90.

[35] Duckett J. W. MAGPI (meatoplasty and glanduloplasty): A procedure for subcoronal hypospadias. *Urol Clin North Am* 1991; 8: 513-9.

[36] Wacksman J. Modification of the onestage flip-flap procedure to repair distal penile hypospadias. *Urol Clin North Am* 1991; 8: 527-30.

[37] Koff S. A., Mobilization of the urethra in the surgical treatment of hypospadias. *J Urol* 1981; 125: 394-7.

[38] Spencer J. R., Perlmutter A. D. Sleeve advancement distal hypospadias repair. *J Urol* 1990; 144: 523-5.

[39] Duckett J. W., The island flap technique for hypospadias repair. *Urol Clin Noth Am* 1981; 8: 503-11.

[40] Devine C. J., Horton C. E., Hypospadias repair. *J Urol* 1977; 118:188-93.

[41] Smith E. D. Durham Smith repair of hypospadias. *Urol Clin North Am* 1981; 8: 451-5.

[42] Greenfield S. P., Sadler P. T., Wan J. Two stage repair for severe hypospadias. *J Urol* 1994; 152: 498-501.

[43] Horton C. E., Devine C. J., Graham J. K. Fistulas of the penile urethra. *Plast Reconstr Surg* 1980; 66: 407-18.

[44] Duckett J. W. Hypospadias. In Gillenwater J. Y., Grayhack J. T., Howards S. S., Mitchell M. E. eds, *Adult and Pediatric Urology,* St Louis: Mosby Year Book, 1991: 2103-39.

[45] Kaya C., Bektic J., Radmayr C., Schwentner C., Bartsch G., Oswald J. The efficacy of dihydrotestosterone transdermal gel before primary hypospadias surgery: A prospective, controlled, randomized study. *J Urol* 2008; 179: 684-8.

[46] Meir D. B., Livne P. M. Is prophylactic antimicrobial treatment necessary after hypospadias repair. *J Urol* 2004; 171: 2621-2.

[47] Ulman I., Erikçi V., Avano lu A., Gökdemir A. The effect of suturing technique and material complication rate following hypospadias repair. *Eur J Pediatr Surg* 1997; 7: 156-7.

[48] Elbakry A. Management of urethrocutaneous fistula after hypospadias repair: 10 years' experience. *BJU Int* 2001; 88: 590-5.

[49] Hayashi Y., Mogami M., Kojima Y. et al., Results of closure of urethrocutaneous fistulas after hypospadias repair. *Int J Urol* 1998; 5: 167-9.

[50] Shankar K. R., Losty P. D., Hopper M., Wong L., Rickwood A. M. Outcome of hypospadias fistula repair. *BJU Int* 2002; 89: 103–5.

[51] Simon H. K., McLario D. J., Bruns T. B., Zempsky W. T., Wood R. J., Sullivan K. M. Long-term appearance of lacerations repaired using a tissue adhesive. *Pediatrics* 1997; 99: 193-5.

[52] Jain S. K., Kaza R. C., Pahwa M., Bansal S. Role of cyanoacrylate in the management of low fistula in ano: A prospective study. *Int J Colorectal Dis* 2008; 23: 355-8.

[53] Barillari P., Basso L., Larcinese A., Gozzo P., Indinnimeo M. Cyanoacrylate glue in the treatment of ano-rectal fistulas. *Int J Colorectal Dis* 2006; 21: 791-4.

[54] Maluf-Filho F., Sakai P., Ishioka S., Matuguma M. E. Endoscopic sclerosis versus cyanoacrylate endoscopic injection for the first episode of variceal bleeding: A prospective, controlled, and randomized study in Child-Pugh class C patients. *Endoscopy* 2001; 33: 421-7.

[55] Zafar F., Thompson J. N., Pati J., Kiely E. A., Abel P. D. Sutureless circumcision. *Br J Surg* 1993; 80: 859.

[56] Rosin D., Rosenthal R. J., Kuriansky J., Brasesco O., Shabtai M., Ayalon A. Closure of laparoscopic trocar site wounds with cyanoacrilate tissue glue: A simple technical solution. *J Laparoendosc Adv Surg Tech A* 2001; 11: 157-9.

[57] Lapointe S. P., N-Fékété C., Lortat-Jacob S. Early closure of fistula after hypospadias surgery using *n*-butyl-cyanoacrylate: Preliminary results. *J Urol* 2002; 168: 1751-3.

[58] Sinha S., Naik M., Wright V., Timmons J., Campbell A. C. A single blind, prospective, randomized trial comparing *n*-butyl 2-cyanoacrylate tissue adhesive (Indermil) and sutures for skin closure in hand surgery. *J Hand Surg Br* 2001; 26: 264-5.

[59] Coulthard P., Worthington H., Esposito M., Elst M., Waes O. J. Tissue adhesives for closure of surgical incisions. *Cochrane Database Syst Rev* 2004; (2): CD004486.

[60] Shapiro A. J., Dinsmore R. C., North J. H. Jr. Tensile strength of wound closure with cyanoacrylate glue. *Am Surg* 2001; 67:1113-5.

[61] Yildiz A., Bertozzi M., Akin M., Appignani A., Prestipino M., Dokucu A. I. Feasibility of a tubularised incised-plate urethroplasty with double de-epithelised dartos flaps in a failed hypospadias repair: A preliminary report. *Afr J Paediatr Surg.* 2012; 9:8-12.

[62] Yıldız A., Bakan V. Comparison of perimeatal-based flap and tubularized incised plate urethroplasty combined with single or double layer dartos fl ap in distal hypospadias. *Urol Int* 2010; 84:265-8.

[63] Borer J. G., Bauer S. B., Peters C. A. et al., Tubularized incised plate urethroplasty: Expanded use in primary and repeat surgery for hypospadias. *J Urol* 2001; 165:581-5.

[64] Snodgrass W., Lorenzo A. Tubularized incised-plate urethroplasty for hypospadias reoperation. *BJU Int* 2002; 89:98-100.

[65] Yiğiter M., Yildiz A., Oral A., Salman A. B. A comparative study to evaluate the effect of double dartos fl aps in primary hypospadias repair: No fistula anymore. *Int Urol Nephrol* 2010; 42:985-90.

In: Hypospadias
Editor: Daniel H. Preston

ISBN: 978-1-63482-023-3

Chapter 5

Elastosonography of the Corpus Spongiosum: Comparison between Normal and Hypospadic Anatomy

Nicola Zampieri[1], Costanza Bruno[2], Silvia Zambaldo[2] and Francesco Saverio Camoglio[1]*

[1]Department of Surgical Sciences, Paediatric Surgery Unit, University of Verona, Policlinico G. B. Rossi, Verona, Italy

[2]Department of Radiology, University of Verona, Policlinico G. B. Rossi, Verona, Italy

Abstract

Introduction: Elastosonography analyzes the variable elasticity of a tissue by recording the changes of RF pulses from a structure, before and after manual compression.

* Correspondence to: Nicola Zampieri, MD, PhD, Pediatric Surgical Unit, Policlinico "G.B. Rossi", Piazzale L.A. Scuro, 37134 Verona, Italy. E-mail: dr.zampieri@libero.it, Telephone: +39.045.8074916, Fax: +39.045.8074672

The aim of this study is to apply the elastosonography on normal and hypospadic penis to verify the structural differences in tissues composition and stiffness.

Materials and Methods: 60 subjects were enrolled, mean age 24 months: 38 patients on post-operative follow-up for distal hypospadia and 22 age-matched subjects as control group (11 patients waiting for surgery and 11 patients without hypospadias). Elastosonography recorded antero-posterior and transverse diameters of the cavernous corpora, urethral and corpus spongiosum diameters, elastographic index of elasticity of the corpus spongiosum. The latter was defined as soft, medium-hard or hard. We assigned the value 1 to soft tissue, 2 and 3 to medium-hard and hard respectively. All scan were performed at the base of the penis, as far as possible from the region involved in the surgical procedure.

Results: Average antero-posterior and transverse diameters of the cavernous corpora were 4.2 mm (DS 0.83) and 6.5 mm (DS 1.12) for hypospadic group and 7.3 mm (DS 1.28) and 9.0 mm (DS 1.67) for control group. These data showed statistically significant difference between the two groups for both the diameters ($p<0.05$). Corpus spongiosum diameter was 1.9 (DS 0.33) for hypospadic group and 2.7 mm (DS 0.73) for control group ($p<0.05$). Less stiffness after surgery due to the chordee resection. Elastography showed a corpus spongiosum stiffness defined as medium-hard or hard in all cases of the pathologic group and soft in all the subjects of the control group ($p<0.05$).

No significant difference was found for urethra diameter between the two groups.

Conclusions: Elastosonography showed how the hypospadia anatomy is deeply altered, even in an anatomical area far from meatal abnormality: corpus spongiosum in hypospadic penis seems to be globally stiffer and less elastic. Moreover, cavernous corpora are less developed. These results could be used for pre-operative counseling. These preliminary results suggest the feasibility of the elastosonography for the evaluation of hypospadic penis. It could be useful during surgical plan to have a better definition of the calibers and quality of the tissues, especially in proximal hypospadia. We believe that this methodic could also be important during the early post-operative follow-up.

Keywords: Hypospadias; elastosonography; children; treatment

Introduction

For centuries clinicians used palpation to evaluate organs; now, after exploring almost all different methods of interaction of ultrasound, x-ray and magnetic fields with tissue in order to express anatomical maps, interest is arising in evaluating mechanical properties of tissues, i.e. viscoelastic characteristics. This is the field of the so-called tissue strain Imaging techniques, while the term "sonoelastography" is usually used to describe the techniques using steady state excitation methods (see below).

Generally speaking they work in a similar way: information is obtained through the application of a force inducing a modification to a tissue which is closely related to its elasticity. The way information concerning elasticity are expressed is different; it can be either a color or a gray-scale map or it can be a number.

A first classification can be made considering the Imaging technique used to measure tissue displacements: most methods are ultrasound-based techniques but magnetic resonance can be used as well.

A. Us-Based Methods

Two main techniques belong to this group: quasi-static and dynamic methods. In the former methods the distribution of the elastic modulus of the target tissue is inferred through the observation of stress and strain, in the latter through the velocity of the shear waves generated in the tissue [1].

1 - Quasi-static methods share a similar way of working and a similar way of analyzing data. Accurate and precise estimation of the local displacements of tissue with high spatial resolution and high signal-to-noise ratio is required [2]. To deduce elasticity from stress and strain, in these methods a known stimulus is applied to the target, radio-frequency data are collected and compared to pre-stimolation data (Figure 1) using different algorithms – the simpliest being the classical time-delay technique then evolved to more complicated cross-correlation algorithm [3]. The cross-correlation algorithm between post and pre-compression A-lines is used to obtain an estimation of the local strain (Figure 1). The stress is evaluated considering the applied stress vs. the theoretical stress distribution, in order to obtain an estimation of the local axial stress [4]. Stress/strain gives the local Young's modulus, which can be expressed as elastogram (Figure 2). One of the problems when dealing with quasi-static methods is that the target tissue must be locally homogeneous because boundaries can have marked effects on the distribution of applied stresses and this can make it problematic to quantitatively image them, giving rise to inaccurate results. Quasi-static methods can be divided in three categories considering the stimulus which can be applied to the tissue [1-5].

a) *Low-frequency excitation*: in this category are found those methods utilizing low-frequency deformation (on the order of 1-10 Hz) to perturb tissue. Since the frequencies are low they do not generate shear waves and can be considered quasi-static in nature.
b) *Steady state excitation*: techniques using a steady state excitation using the ultrasound transducer represent some of the most commonly utilized approaches to elastographic imaging. Steady-state quasi-static deformations have been applied using either under stepper motor control (with the transducer held in a fixture) or freehand compression using the transducer. This is the most-frequently use method of tissue excitation and is usually referred as "sonoelastography".
c) *Steady state physiological excitation*: physiological stimuli due to respiratory, cardiac muscle deformations and cardiovascular sources have been used for elastographic imaging. Physiological deformation sources, however, introduce challenges due to non-uniform deformations caused and need for gating of the data to obtain reproducible results.

2 - Dynamic methods are based on the detection and tracking of shear waves resulting from mechanical vibration of the tissue. The algorithm used is the "time to peak algorithm" [6]. The main problem consisting with dynamic methods is that the shear waves undergo rapid attenuation. Two main categories can be identified, on the basis of the applied stimulus:

a) *External methods (*i.e., *Transient Elastography)*: a mechanical push from a piston is used to launch a compression wave into the tissue. The transient distortion of the tissue generates a shear wave that travels laterally away from the line of the compression push in a three-dimensional pattern and the movements of the tissue are visualized by an interrogating ultrasound beam. This produces a line on the monitoring screen whose slope indicates the speed of movement of the shear wave which is related to the Young's modulus.
b) *Internal methods (*i.e., *Acoustic Radiation Force Imaging Technique; Supersonic Shear Wave Elastography)*: after selecting a range of interest on a gray-scale map an acoustic push pulse is focused directly to it, inducing the generation of the shear waves. The shear waves travel perpendicular to the ultrasonic beam and undergo a rapid attenuation. But before it happens tracking beams are sent to the tissue, parallel to the main axis, continuously until the passing shear

wavefront is detected. Different algorithms are used to calculate the shear wave velocity (SWV) and thus the elastic modulus [6].

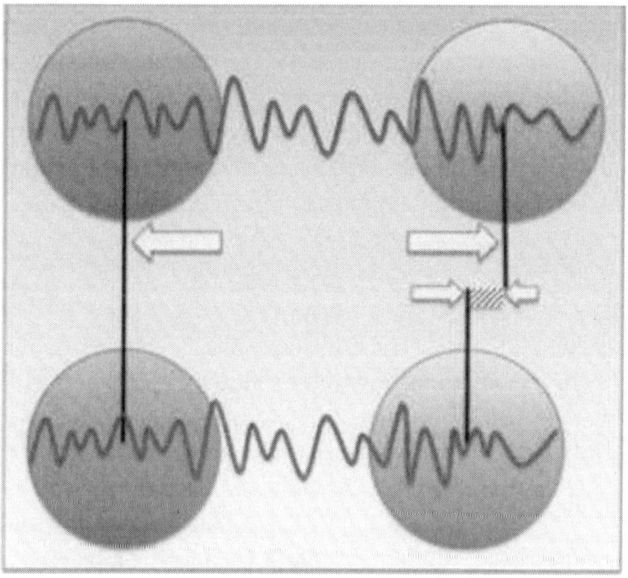

Figure 1. cross-correlation algorithm between post and pre-compression A-lines is used to obtain an estimation of the local strain.

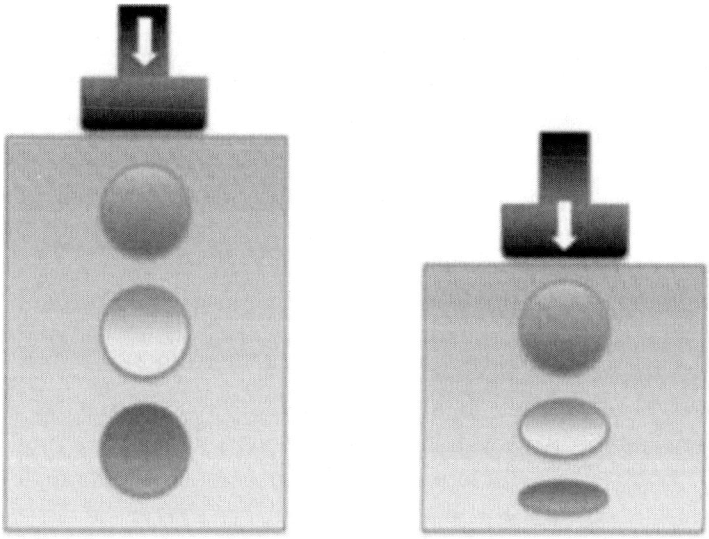

Figure 2. Elastogram and modification during compression.

B. Magnetic Resonance-Based Methods

The principle of MR elastography is very similar to that of sonoelastography. High-frequency vibrations are applied externally to the tissue to induce the generation of shear waves. Tissue displacements are then correlated with the phase shift of the magnetic resonance signals and data are then processed to relate these displacements to mechanical properties. Several factors can affect the results obtained using MR-based elastography, including the frequency of tissue excitation, tissue temperature and the direction of wave propagation and polarization.

Hypospadias and Basic Pathology

The formation of fibrous scar in the tunica albuginea of the phallus is referred to as chronic inflammation of the tunica albuginea like in the common Peyronie's disease. The fibrosis or the fibrous tissue are usually detectable as an indurated plaque by palpation or by radiographic findings. In hypospadias penile curvature is sometimes present without a palpable plaque. Ultrasound is the primary imaging technique in the evaluation of Peyronie's penile pathology and has a role in demonstrating calcifications in lesions and, with duplex studies, identifying potential concomitant vascular compromise. Case series in Peyronie's disease have reported the detection of penile plaques with B-mode ultrasonography in 39% to 97% of cases. [7]

Sonoelastography (tissue elasticity imaging) is an emerging ultrasound modality designed to evaluate the stiffness of biological tissues and allows inferences to be made about pathology in the same manner as palpation. Sonoelastography uses ultrasonic techniques to determine differences in relative tissue elasticity, a measure of tissue stiffness (also known as Young's modulus). When a compressive stress is placed on tissue, a degree of deformation (strain) occurs. The amount of deformation is inversely proportional to the stiffness of the tissue. Furthermore, the amount of stress required to deform the tissue is directly proportional to the stiffness of the tissue.

There are two modalities that are frequently used to induce stress in a tissue with ultrasound. Real-time sonoelastography employs manual compression of the tissue with the ultrasound probe to produce a stress on the tissue. If the tissue has a uniform stiffness, then the strain is uniform. If there is a variable elasticity of the tissue, then there will be variations in the strain that can be detected by the ultrasound probe. Real-time sonoelastography takes advantage of variations in the tissue deformation in this way to demonstrate the relative differences in tissue stiffness. These differences are displayed with a color scale overlying their location on the ultrasound image. Shear wave sonoeslastography enlists another type of stress, shear stress, to determine elasticity [8]. Shear stress arises when a surface of a material is subjected to stress in a direction parallel to that surface and the opposite surface is held in place by an opposing force. A stress induced at a certain location in tissue will deform the tissue in that location and, because the tissue around it is held in place by the opposing force of friction and normal forces of adjacent tissue structure, a shear stress is generated. The shear stress can also propagate radially from the location of its source through the surrounding tissue in the same manner as waves propagate radially away from the site where a pebble hits the surface of a body of water. These waves are shear waves. The tissue deformations generated by these waves can be detected by ultrasound receivers with very fast acquisition speeds [9, 10]. The ultrasound transducers are uniquely constructed to generate these shear wave but also can be used for more traditional diagnostic ultrasound. The speed at which shear waves propagate is inversely proportional to the square root of the medium's density and directly proportional to the square root of its elasticity. Thus, the more stiff (the greater the shear modulus), the faster the shear waves travel. It is this relationship and the notion that tissue density has little variability within an organ that allow the stiffness of tissue to be determined by calculation of the speed of shear wave propagation through the tissue. This is the principle employed in shear wave sonoelastography to determine elasticity. The sonoelastographic images may demonstrate changes in the tissue that extend beyond those that can be demonstrated on B-mode ultrasound. Specifically, there is a potential with sonoelastography to demonstrate changes not simply limited to the tunica albuginea but also to the cavernosal body as well. The application of this technology to clinical practice is currently limited by its relatively limited availability compared with B-mode ultrasonography. Penile Sonoelastography in cases of hypospadias might be useful to identify fibrosis area and anatomical and physiological condition of tissue before surgery.

Case Series and Personal Experience with Elastonosography

During the period January 2010 and January 2014 60 subjects were enrolled, mean age 24 months: 38 patients on post-operative follow-up for distal hypospadia and 22 age-matched subjects as control group (11 patients waiting for surgery and 11 patients without hypospadias). Elastosonography recorded antero-posterior and transverse diameters of the cavernous corpora, urethral and corpus spongiosum diameters, elastographic index of elasticity of the corpus spongiosum. The latter was defined as soft, medium-hard or hard. We assigned the value 1 to soft tissue, 2 and 3 to medium-hard and hard respectively. With standard ultrasound we recorded all bladder characteristics (bladder neck thickness, detrusor thickness and bladder capacity).

All scan were performed by the same radiologist at the base of the penis, as far as possible from the region involved in the surgical procedure.

Sonoelastography was used in the evaluation of fibrosis in the corpus spongiosum and in the corpus cavernosum. We used a linear probe ultrasonograph (US) (Esaote Gold Platform MayLab 60, Genoa, Italy) equipped with elasto software (ElaXto, Esaote). First B-mode images were obtained for each penis. Afterwards ES was performed by applying light vertical pressure followed by decompression until a good-quality image was obtained. The elastogram based on a color scale was displayed on the B-mode image which ranges from green to blu. Green represented tissue with greatest elastic strain meaning softest components, while blu represented tissue with no strain meaning hardest components. The elasticity scores were classified into 3 score. Results were expressed using an expressed through a semiquantitative 3-point scale where 1 represents more elastic tissue (predominantly green and red) and 3 represent less elastic tissue (predominantly blue). 2 is an intermediate class where blue and green are mixed.

During the study we recorded: patients data (date of birth, age at surgery), type of hypospadias and malformations associated, presence of chordee and surgical procedure used (technique, stiches, tube) and complications at 3 and 6 months.

Oral and written consent was obtained by each parents and the study was approved by internal IRB. The ultrasound study was performed in two different manners: longitudinal and transverse way. The transverse mode identified proximal to distal part of the penis while the longitudinal one was used to evaluate corporus cavernosum and corpus spongiosum and arterial supply. During the penile ultrasound we evaluated : urethral thickness, corpus cavernosum diameter, corpus cavernosum angle and corpus spongiosum thickness.

Results

Average antero-posterior and transverse diameters of the cavernous corpora were 4.2 mm (DS 0.83) and 6.5 mm (DS 1.12) for hypospadic group and 7.3 mm (DS 1.28) and 9.0 mm (DS 1.67) for control group. These data showed statistically significant difference between the two groups for both the diameters ($p<0.05$).

Corpus spongiosum diameter was 1.9 (DS 0.33) for hypospadic group and 2.7 mm (DS 0.73) for control group ($p<0.05$). Less stiffness after surgery due to the chordee resection.

Elastosonography showed a corpus spongiosum stiffness defined as medium-hard or hard in all cases of the pathologic group and soft in all the subjects of the control group ($p<0.05$).(figure 3-7).

No significant difference was found for urethra diameter between the two groups (post surgical group and controls).

This data could demonstrate that surgical procedure doesn't affect urethral diameter and that after surgery urethral diameter is similar respect to non hypospadic penis.

The detrusor thickness and stiffness evaluations showed that patients with hypospadias not still treated had a stiffer muscle than controls and treated patients; this data could be explained with a physiological/pathological condition related to the anomalous external urethral meatus.

This data is not confirmed measuring the bladder neck thickness where there was not a statistical differences between groups.

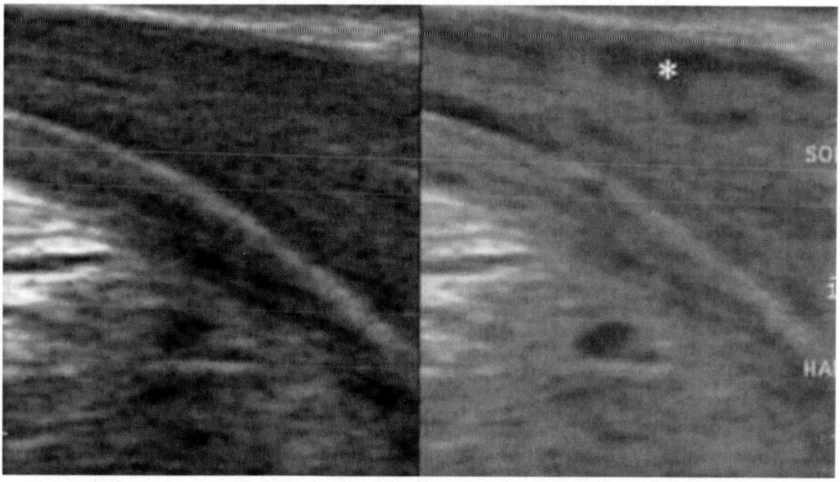

Figure 3. Case 1: proximal hypospadias - see fibrosis and the "blu" of corpus cavernosum at the penile base.

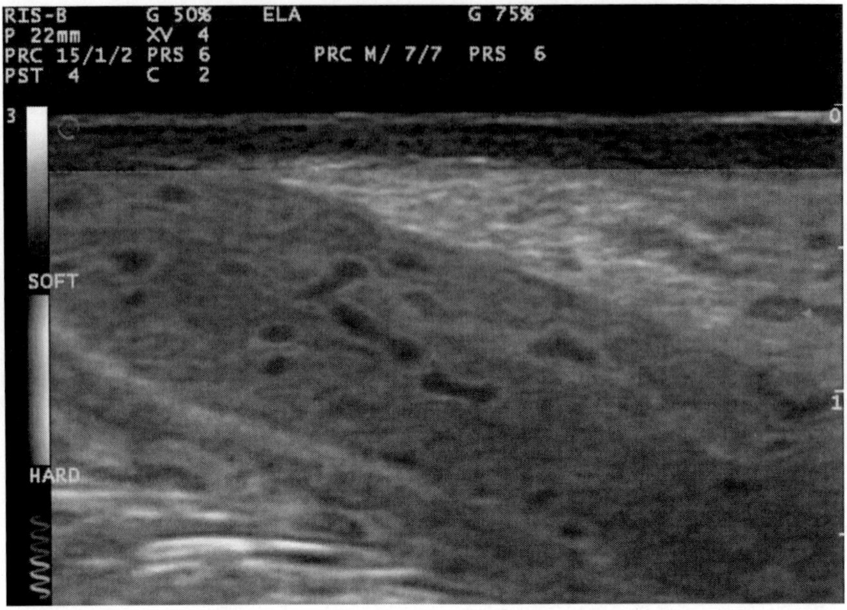

Figure 4. Case 2: normal penis 1: - see "green" and "red" all around the urethra and the penile base.

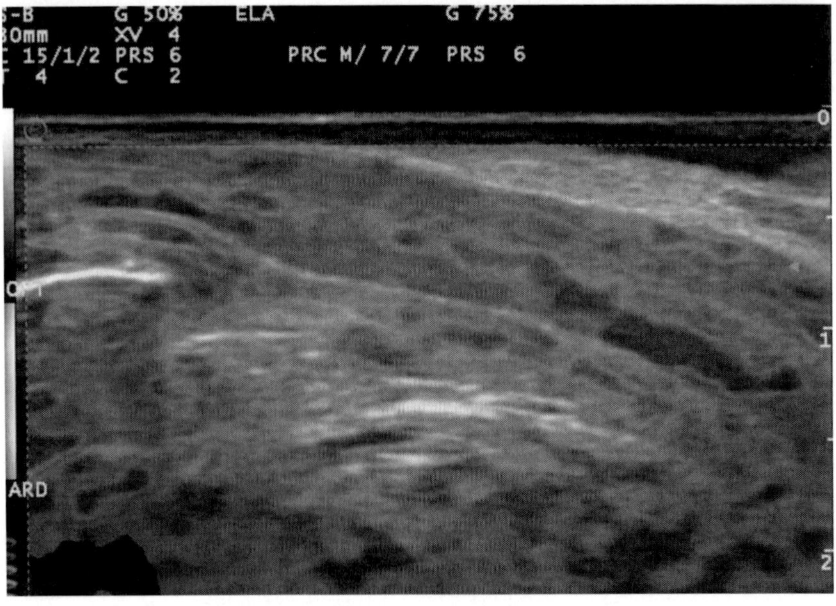

Figure 5. Case 3: normal penis 2 - "red" expression of normal tissue all aournd the corpus cavernosum.

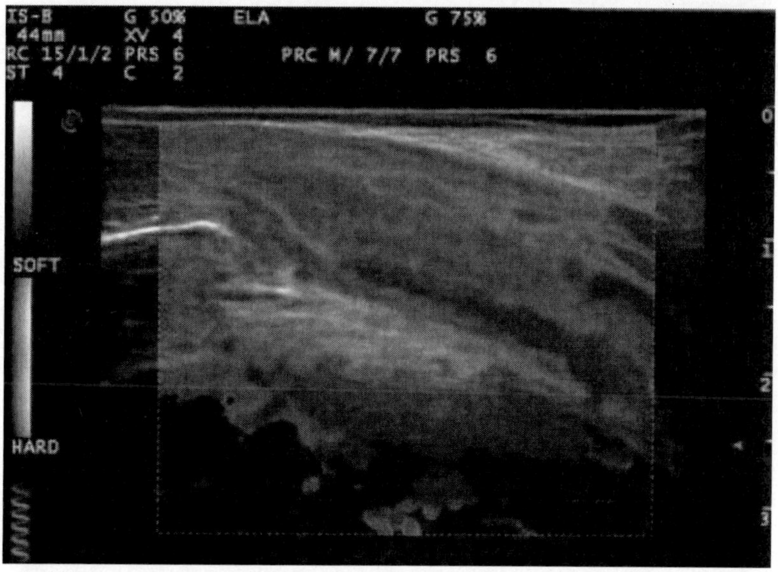

Figure 6. Case 4: distal hypospadias - pre-surgical view: see fibrosis near the urethra (in the middle and at the penile base); see glans defect at the top

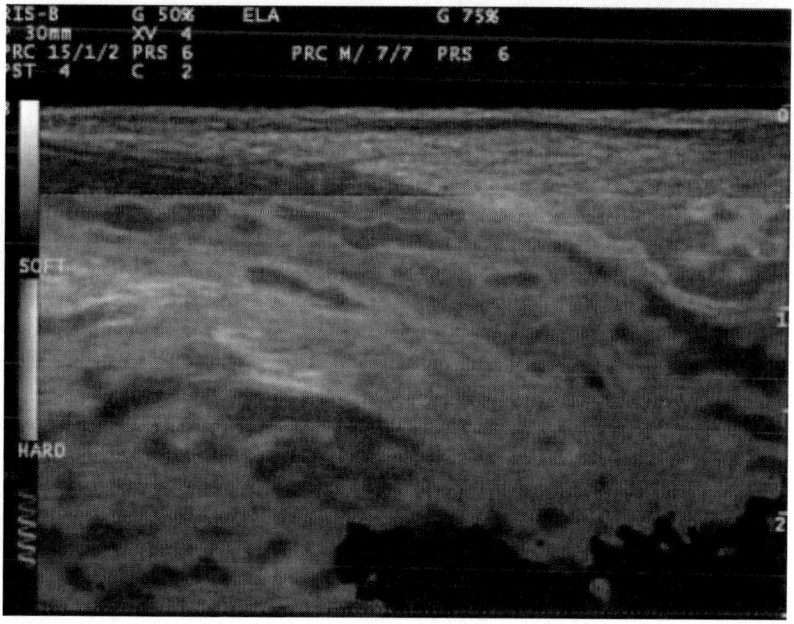

Figure 7. Case 4: post-op view (see less stiffness near the urethra and near the corpus cavernosum); see the "normal" glans closure at the top.

Evaluation of corpus spongiosum diameters showed a statistical differences between groups: patients with hypospadias (treated and untreated) had smaller corpus spongiosum respect to controls. This mean that hypospadias is not only an urethral malformation. This data is also confirmed during the evaluation of the corpus cavernosum.

Studing the angle between both corpus cavernosum the results are intresting: there is a statistical differences between groups especially between non treated patients with hypospadias and controls; elastosonography showed that untreated patients had hard stiffness of corpus cavernosum and the angle is higher respect to controls and treated patients respectively.

Discussion

Sonoelastography is an imaging technique useful to know the elasticity of tissue; results are expressed following a color scale where in red are well vascularized tissue with a good elasticity, and blu are stiffer tissue. Green colour represent a mixed stiffness.

The useful of this technique represent the capacity of real-time ultrasound to evaluate tissue and the stiffness of tissue immediatly during the examination, focusing on a specific site or area. The hard stiffness in hypospadic penis represent the outcome of this procedure; hypospadias is not an urethral disease alone but there are many components. There are less elasticity of corpus spongiosum and cavernosum with an higher angle between corpus cavernosum. This mean that is essential to evaluate during surgery all these aspects; Fibrosis is in the ventral part of the penis all around the urethra and near the proximal urethra where the corpus cavernosum divided and the angle is greater.

In our study there was not a statistical difference between penile lenght between groups, but this result can be found especially between treated patients and controls.

Pre-Operative Counseling Value of Elastosonography

There are many different technique for hypospadias repair.

The choice is based on different factors but usually type of hypospadias, glans appearance, quality of tissues, presence of chordee and surgeon experience seems to be the most used.

The real uretral meatus position represent the first consideration point for which surgical technique should be used, but during surgery, after the total penile exposition, some cases are not as suspected and the technique should be re-evaluate. Also for urethral wall, during surgery many of the coronal hypospadias are different after the toal penile exposition and the "real" urethra with good tissue is more proximal than expected. The presence of chordee is another important point during surgery; to have a good functional results all chordee or scaring tissue should be removed especially near the new urethra.

It is for this reason that ultrasound and elastosonography might be useful to plan the surgical procedures in term of scaring tissue, chordee, vascularization of tissue, "real" meatal position, real urethral wall, angle of corpus cavernosum in oreder to reduce complication and to have the best surgical reconstruction.

Considerations

This is a cromatic measure of stiffness and elasticity of different tissues. Results are expressed with different colors (green, red, blue) and the interpretation is essential. This is a real time procedure, and results could be different after time. There is not literature about hypospadias and elastosonography and this is a limit but probably is the essential point to consider this method in the future.

Post surgical follow-up in this patients is important especially for parents; but a correct and well done pre-surgical counseling could reduce complications and parents anxiety.

Conclusion

Elastosonography showed how the hypospadia anatomy is deeply altered, even in an anatomical area far from meatal abnormality: corpus spongiosum in hypospadic penis seems to be globally stiffer and less elastic. Moreover, cavernous corpora are less developed. These results could be used for pre-operative counseling.

References

[1] Li Y, Snedeker JG. Elastography: modality-specific approaches, clinical applications, and research horizons. *Skeletal Radiol.* 2011 Apr;40(4):389-97.

[2] Varghese T. Quasi-Static Ultrasound Elastography. *Ultrasound Clin.* 2009 Jul;4(3):323-338.

[3] Hall TJ. AAPM/RSNA physics tutorial for residents: topics in US: beyond the basics: elasticity imaging with US. *Radiographics.* 2003 Nov-Dec;23(6):1657-*71 Phys. Med. Biol.*2000 Jun;45(6):1423-35.

[4] Ophir J, Garra B, Kallel F, Konofagou E, Krouskop T, Righetti R, Varghese T. Elastographic imaging. *Ultrasound Med. Biol.* 2000 May;26 Suppl 1:S23-9.

[5] Pesavento A,Lorenz A,Siebers S,Ermert H. New real-time strain imaging concepts using diagnostic ultrasound. *Ultrasound Clin.* 2009 Jul;4(3):323-338.

[6] Nightingale. Acoustic radiation force imaging: a review. *Curr. Med. Imaging Rev.* 2011 Nov 1; 7(4): 328-339.

[7] Richards G, Goldenberg E, Pek H, Gilbert BR. Penile sonoelastography for the localization of a non-palpable non sonographically visualized lesion in a patient with penile curvature from Peyronie's disease. *J. Sex Med.* 11: 516-520; 2014.

[8] Lopez JA, Jarow JP. Duplex ultrasound findings in men with Peyronie's disease. *Urol Radiol.* 12:199-202; 1999.

[9] Bamber JC. Ultrasound elasticity imaging: definition and technology. *Eur. Radiol.* 9; S327-330; 1999.

[10] Wells PNT, Liang HD. Medical ultrasound imaging of soft tissue strain and elasticity. *J. R. Soc. interface* 8; 1521-1549; 2011.

Index

#

A

B

C

D

E

F

G

K

L

M

N

R

S

T

U

V

W

X